Handbook of
Urticaria

Handbook of Urticaria

An Initiative of GA²LEN Urticaria Centers of Reference and Excellence (UCARE)

Editor

Kiran V Godse MD PhD FRCP (Glasgow)
Department of Dermatology
Dr DY Patil Medical College
Navi Mumbai, Maharashtra, India

Associate Editors

Abhishek De MD FAGE MRCP-SCE (Dermatology)
Department of Dermatology
Calcutta National Medical College
Kolkata, West Bengal, India

Anant Patil MD
Department of Pharmacology
Dr DY Patil Medical College
Navi Mumbai, Maharashtra, India

Foreword

Torsten Zuberbier
Marcus Maurer
Ana Maria Giménez-Arnau

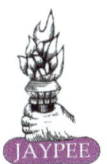

JAYPEE BROTHERS MEDICAL PUBLISHERS
The Health Sciences Publisher
New Delhi | London

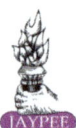 **Jaypee Brothers Medical Publishers (P) Ltd**

Headquarters
EMCA House
23/23-B, Ansari Road, Daryaganj
New Delhi 110 002, India
Landline: +91-11-23272143, +91-11-23272703
+91-11-23282021, +91-11-23245672
E-mail: jaypee@jaypeebrothers.com

Corporate Office
Jaypee Brothers Medical Publishers (P) Ltd.
4838/24, Ansari Road, Daryaganj
New Delhi 110 002, India
Phone: +91-11-43574357
Fax: +91-11-43574314
E-mail: jaypee@jaypeebrothers.com

Overseas Office
JP Medical Ltd.
83, Victoria Street, London
SW1H 0HW (UK)
Phone: +44-20 3170 8910
Fax: +44(0)20 3008 6180
E-mail: info@jpmedpub.com

Website: www.jaypeebrothers.com
Website: www.jaypeedigital.com

© 2022, Jaypee Brothers Medical Publishers

The views and opinions expressed in this book are solely those of the original contributor(s)/author(s) and do not necessarily represent those of editor(s) of the book.

All rights reserved by the author. No part of this publication may be reproduced, stored or transmitted in any form or by any means, electronic, mechanical, photocopying, recording or otherwise, without the prior permission in writing of the publishers.

All brand names and product names used in this book are trade names, service marks, trademarks or registered trademarks of their respective owners. The publisher is not associated with any product or vendor mentioned in this book.

Medical knowledge and practice change constantly. This book is designed to provide accurate, authoritative information about the subject matter in question. However, readers are advised to check the most current information available on procedures included and check information from the manufacturer of each product to be administered, to verify the recommended dose, formula, method and duration of administration, adverse effects and contraindications. It is the responsibility of the practitioner to take all appropriate safety precautions. Neither the publisher nor the author(s)/editor(s) assume any liability for any injury and/or damage to persons or property arising from or related to use of material in this book.

This book is sold on the understanding that the publisher is not engaged in providing professional medical services. If such advice or services are required, the services of a competent medical professional should be sought.

Every effort has been made where necessary to contact holders of copyright to obtain permission to reproduce copyright material. If any have been inadvertently overlooked, the publisher will be pleased to make the necessary arrangements at the first opportunity. The **CD/DVD-ROM** (if any) provided in the sealed envelope with this book is complimentary and free of cost. **It is Not meant for sale**.

Inquiries for bulk sales may be solicited at: jaypee@jaypeebrothers.com

*Handbook of Urticaria / **Kiran V Godse***

First Edition: **2022**

ISBN: 978-93-5465-026-0

Contributors

EDITOR

Kiran V Godse
Department of Dermatology
Dr DY Patil Medical College
Navi Mumbai, Maharashtra, India

ASSOCIATE EDITORS

Abhishek De
Department of Dermatology
Calcutta National Medical College
Kolkata, West Bengal, India

Anant Patil
Department of Pharmacology
Dr DY Patil Medical College
Navi Mumbai, Maharashtra, India

CONTRIBUTING AUTHORS

Abhishek De
Department of Dermatology
Calcutta National Medical College
Kolkata, West Bengal, India

Agnieszka Sikora
European Center for Diagnosis and
Treatment of Urticaria (GA²LEN UCARE
Network), Medical University of Silesia in
Katowice, Poland

Alicja Kasperska-Zajac
European Center for Diagnosis and
Treatment of Urticaria (GA²LEN UCARE
Network)
Medical University of Silesia in Katowice
Poland

Ana Maria Giménez-Arnau
Dermatology Department
Hospital del Mar, IMIM
Universitat Autònoma de Barcelona

Anant Patil
Department of Pharmacology
Dr DY Patil Medical College
Navi Mumbai, Maharashtra, India

Angèle Soria
Sorbonne Université, Service de
Dermatologie et d'Allergologie, Hôpital
Tenon, Assistance Publique Hôpitaux de
Paris, 4 rue de la Chine 75020 Paris, France
Cimi-Paris, INSERM U1135, Paris, France

Aslı Gelincik
Immunology and Allergic Diseases
Internal Medicine, Istanbul Faculty of
Medicine Istanbul University, Turkey

Carla Ritchie
Allergy and Immunology Section
Hospital Italiano
Buenos Aires, Argentina

Connor Prosty
Faculty of Medicine
McGill University
Montreal, QC, Canada

Célia Costa
Immunoallergology Department
Hospital de Santa Maria
Centro Hospitalar Universitário Lisboa
Norte EPE, Lisbon, Portugal

Contributors

Daria Fomina
Moscow Center of Allergy and Immunology
Clinical State Hospital 52, Moscow Ministry of Healthcare
Department of Clinical Immunology and Allergology
First Moscow State University(Sechenov University), Russian Federation

Désirée Larenas-Linnemann
Center of Excellence in Asthma and Allergy
Médica Sur Clinical Foundation and Hospital
México City, Mexico

Elena Netchiporouk
Division of Dermatology
McGill University Health Centre
Montreal, QC, Canada

Emek Kocatürk
Department of Dermatology
Koç University School of Medicine
Istanbul, Turkey

Germán Darío Ramón
Instituto de Alergia e Inmunologia del Sur., Bahia Blanca, Argentina; Hospital Italiano Regional del Sur., Allergy Section
Bahia Blanca, Argentina

Gordon Sussman
University of Toronto
Toronto, ON, Canada

Guillet Carole
Allergy Unit
Department of Dermatology
University Hospital Zurich
Zurich, Switzerland
Medical Faculty, University of Zurich
Zurich, Switzerland
Dermatological Allergology
Department of Dermatology
Charité – Universitätsmedizin Berlin
Berlin, Germany

Hassan Mobayed
Allergy and Immunology Section
Hamad Medical Corporation
Doha, Qatar

Hermenio Lima
Lima's Excellence in Allergy and Dermatology Research (LEADER) Director
Associate Professor Division of Dermatology and Allergy and Clinical Immunology
Division Director of Dermatology
Department of Medicine, Michael G. DeGroote School of Medicine
McMaster University, Hamilton, ON

I Boccon-Gibod
National Reference Center for Angioedema (CREAK)
Department of Clinical Immunology
Grenoble University Hospital
Grenoble, France

Iman Hamed Nasr
Immunology and Allergy Unit
Internal Medicine Department
Royal Hospital, Oman

Iris Medina
Consultant Specialist Allergy and Clinical Immunology, Department of Allergy
Centro Médico Vitae, Av. San Martín 966
9 de Julio, Argentina

Ismahaan Abdisalaam
Department of Dermatology
Erasmus Medical Center, Rotterdam, The Netherlands; Centre for Human Drug Research, Leiden, The Netherlands

Ivan Cherrez Ojeda
Allergy, Immunology and Pulmonary Medicine, Medical and Research Director of Respiralab, Research Professor at Espiritu Santo University (UEES), Respiralab, Clinica Kennedy, Seccion Delta, Av 9na. Oeste y Av. San Jorge, Ecuador

Jesper Grønlund Holm
Department of Dermatology
Bispebjerg Hospital, Copenhagen, Denmark

Jonathan A Bernstein
University of Cincinnati
Department of Internal Medicine
Division of Immunology
Allergy Section, University of Cincinnati
231 Albert Sabin Way, ML#563
Cincinnati, OH

Jorge Sanchez
Group of Clinical and Experimental Allergy
IPSU Clinic
University of Antioquia (Medellín, Colombia)

Kanokvalai Kulthanan
Department of Dermatology
Faculty of Medicine Siriraj Hospital
Mahidol University
2 Wanglang Road, Bangkoknoi
Bangkok 10700, Thailand

Kiran V Godse
Department of Dermatology
Dr DY Patil Medical College
Navi Mumbai, Maharashtra, India

Krzysztof Rutkowski
Department of Allergy
Guy's and St Thomas' Hospital and Urticaria
Clinic, St John's Institute of Dermatology
London, United Kingdom

L Bouillet
National Reference Center for
Angioedema (CREAK)
Department of Clinical Immunology
Grenoble University Hospital
Grenoble, France

Leonor Esteves Caldeira
Immunoallergology Department
Hospital de Santa Maria
Centro Hospitalar Universitário Lisboa Norte
EPE, Lisbon, Portugal

Leu Noemi
Allergy Unit, Department of Dermatology
University Hospital Zurich
Zurich, Switzerland
Medical Faculty, University of Zurich
Zurich, Switzerland

L Karla Arruda
Ribeirao Preto Medical School
University of Sao Paulo, Brazil

Luis Felipe Ensina
Federal University of São Paulo
São Paulo, Brazil

Magdalena Zając
European Center for Diagnosis and
Treatment of Urticaria (GA2LEN UCARE
Network), Medical University of Wroclaw,
Poland

Maia Gotua
David Tvildiani Medical University
Center of Allergy and Immunology
Tbilisi, Georgia

Margarida Gonçalo
Clinic of Dermatology
University Hospital and Faculty of Medicine
University of Coimbra
Coimbra, Portugal

Maria Luiza Oliva Alonso
Federal University of Rio de Janeiro
Rio de Janeiro, Brazil

Martijn van Doorn
Department of Dermatology
Erasmus Medical Center, Rotterdam,
the Netherlands; Centre for Human Drug
Research, Leiden, the Netherlands

Maryam Al-Nesf
Allergy and Immunology Section
Hamad Medical Corporation
Doha, Qatar

Michael P Makris
Allergy Unit
2nd Department of Dermatology and
Venereology
Medical School, National and Kapodistrian
University of Athens
Attikon University Hospital
Athens, Greece

Michael Rudenko
London Allergy and Immunology Centre
London, United Kingdom

Michelle Le
Division of Dermatology
McGill University Health Centre
Montreal, QC, Canada

Mojca Bizjak
Division of Allergy
University Clinic of Respiratory and
Allergic Diseases Golnik
Golnik, Slovenia

Mona Al-Ahmad
Microbiology Department
Faculty of Medicine
Kuwait University, Kuwait

CONTRIBUTORS

Moshe Ben-Shoshan
Division of Allergy
Immunology and Dermatology
Montreal Children's Hospital
Montreal, QC, Canada

M Sendhil Kumaran
Department of Dermatology
PGIMER, Chandigarh, India

Naoko Inomata
Department of Environmental Immuno-Dermatology Yokohama City University
Graduate School of Medicine, Japan

Nasseer Masoodi
Ambulatory General Internal Medicine,
Department of Medicine
Hamad Medical Corporation
Doha, Qatar

Nasser Mohammad Porras
Dermatology Department Hospital del Mar,
IMIM, Universitat Autònoma
Barcelona, Spain

Niall Conlon
Department of Immunology
St James's Hospital, Dublin; Department of Clinical Immunology, Trinity College Dublin

Nidhi Sharma
Department of Dermatology
Medanta - The Medicity
Gurugram, Haryana, India

Paulo Ricardo Criado
Centro Universitário FMABC
Santo André, Brazil

Pelin Kuteyla CAN
Department of Dermatology
Bahcesehir University, School of Medicine
Istanbul, Turkey

Ricardo Cardona
Group of Clinical and Experimental Allergy
Faculty of Medecine
University of Antioquia (Medellín, Colombia)

Riccardo Asero
Ambulatorio di Allergologia
Clinica San Carlo
Paderno Dugnano (MI), Italy

Roberta FJ Criado
Centro Universitário FMABC
Santo André, Brazil

Rosana Câmara Agondi
Clinical Immunology and Allergy Division
University of São Paulo
SP, Brazil

Schmid-Grendelmeier Peter
Allergy Unit
Department of Dermatology
University Hospital Zurich
Zurich, Switzerland
Medical Faculty
University of Zurich
Zurich, Switzerland
Christine Kühne Center for Allergy Research and Education CK-CARE
Davos, Switzerland

Semra Demir
Immunology and Allergic Diseases
Internal Medicine
Istanbul Faculty of Medicine
Istanbul University, Turkey

Sergio Duarte Dortas Junior
Federal University of Rio de Janeiro
Rio de Janeiro, Brazil

Silvia Ferrucci
Dermatology Unit
Fondazione IRCCS Ca' Granda Ospedale Maggiore Policlinico
Milan, Italy
Department of Pathophysiology and Transplantation, Università degli Studi di Milano Milan, Italy

Simon Francis Thomsen
Department of Dermatology
Bispebjerg Hospital
Copenhagen, Denmark

Sofianne Gabrielli
Division of Allergy, Immunology and Dermatology
Montreal Children's Hospital
Montreal, QC, Canada

Solange Oliveira Rodrigues Valle
Federal University of Rio de Janeiro
Rio de Janeiro, Brazil

Tessa Niemeyer-van der Kolk
Centre for Human Drug Research
Leiden, the Netherlands

Vignesh Narayan
Department of Dermatology
PGIMER, Chandigarh, India

Foreword

"Urticaria" and "angioedema" are common problems. In many patients, they present as chronic disease with a severe impact on their lives. In fact, most patients with chronic urticaria currently do not have their disease under control. The last years we have seen considerable progress in our understanding of urticaria and angioedema. We now better understand the pathogenesis of the disease, have tools for its management, and, most importantly, effective treatment options. This progress is largely based on what we have learnt from our patients. Our patients have told us about the impact of urticaria, the unmet needs, our gaps of knowledge, and how to improve our management approaches to this disease. We need to continue to listen to our patients and learn from this. This *Handbook of Urticaria* helps with this. The more than 20 chapters written by a total number of 68 authors are based on patients' stories, actual patients' cases from clinical practice as well as physician experience and published evidence.

This *Handbook on Urticaria* would not exist without the global network of Urticaria Centers of Reference and Excellence (UCARE). Most of the authors of the chapters of this book are UCARE members, and much of the information presented in this handbook is from what we have learnt from patients managed by UCAREs, in all parts of the world. The UCARE network aims to increase knowledge of urticaria and to educate physicians who treat patients with urticaria, on a global scale. UCAREs work together in numerous projects, such as the development of this handbook, but also on a global registry study, CURE, as well as scientific projects and educational formats and events. We thank the members of the UCARE network and the authors for their continued dedication and contributions to this book. We are sure this *Handbook on Urticaria* will help to improve patient care and disease management.

This *Handbook on Urticaria* exists because of Kiran Godse. Kiran and his UCARE team are a motor of our network, and we are very grateful to him and his team for the energy and determination invested in this handbook.

We hope that you enjoy the read and benefit from the information presented in this book.

May it help to improve the treatment of urticaria and angioedema worldwide!

The UCARE Steering Committee
**Marcus Maurer, Torsten Zuberbier, Ana Maria Giménez-Arnau,
Kanokvalai Kulthanan, Luis Felipe Ensina**

Preface

I am happy to present *"Handbook of Urticaria"* to the readers. This book is unique in terms of its concept and preparation. The purpose of writing this handbook is to increase awareness about urticaria among family physicians, consultant physicians, and postgraduate students of dermatologists. The book is an initiative of GA²LEN Urticaria Centers of Reference and Excellence (UCARE). Authors from UCARE centers all over the world have contributed chapters in this book. The book contains chapters covering all aspects of urticaria from its presentation to the management.

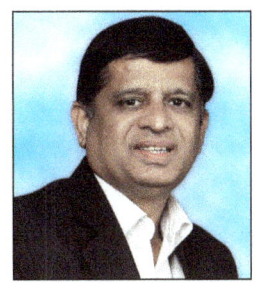

I am sure readers will appreciate the reader-friendly nature of the book because of several clinical images, tables, and figures. I thank the management of DY Patil Hospital, Nerul, Navi Mumbai, Maharashtra, India for constant support in academic endeavors. I also thank Associate Editors, Dr Abhishek De and Dr Anant Patil for their constant support and help in coordinating with authors of all chapters and completing the task of writing the book in time.

I wish to thank my family, Dr Meenal, Dr Gauri, and Atharva for supporting my academics.

Kiran V Godse

Contents

Chapter 1	**Urticaria: Introduction and Classification** Jonathan A Bernstein, Michael P Makris, Germán Darío Ramón	1
Chapter 2	**Etiopathogenesis** Leonor Esteves Caldeira, Célia Costa, Mona Al-Ahmad, Jorge Sanchez, Ricardo Cardona	3
Chapter 3	**Acute Urticaria** Kanokvalai Kulthanan, Angèle Soria, Iris Medina	9
Chapter 4	**Chronic Spontaneous Urticaria** Kiran V Godse, Abhishek De	13
Chapter 5	**Chronic Inducible Urticaria** Pelin Kuteyla CAN, Daria Fomina, Emek Kocatürk	24
Chapter 6	**Angioedema** Niall Conlon, I Boccon-Gibod, L Bouillet	33
Chapter 7	**Urticaria and Comorbidities** Maia Gotua, Rosana Câmara Agondi, Ivan Cherrez Ojeda	38
Chapter 8	**Role of Infections in Urticaria** Michael Rudenko	44
Chapter 9	**Differential Diagnosis** Mojca Bizjak, Krzysztof Rutkowski, Margarida Gonçalo	48
Chapter 10	**Diagnostic Approach** Maryam Al-Nesf, Riccardo Asero, L Karla Arruda	55
Chapter 11	**Patient-reported Outcome Measures** Alicja Kasperska-Zajac, Solange Oliveira Rodrigues Valle, Sergio Duarte Dortas Junior, Agnieszka Sikora, Magdalena Zając, Maria Luiza Oliva Alonso	60
Chapter 12	**Antihistamines** Anant Patil, Gordon Sussman, Nidhi Sharma	65
Chapter 13	**Cyclosporine A** Aslı Gelincik, Semra Demir, Silvia Ferrucci	70

Chapter 14	**Omalizumab** Nasser Mohammad Porras, Luis Felipe Ensina, Ana Maria Giménez-Arnau	72
Chapter 15	**Other Therapeutic Options** Jesper Grønlund Holm, Paulo Ricardo Criado, Roberta F J Criado, Simon Francis Thomsen	79
Chapter 16	**Treatment Algorithm for Chronic Urticaria** Ismahaan Abdisalaam, Tessa Niemeyer-van der Kolk, Désirée Larenas-Linnemann, Martijn van Doorn	84
Chapter 17	**Urticaria in Children** Connor Prosty, Sofianne Gabrielli, Michelle Le, Elena Netchiporouk, Moshe Ben-Shoshan	88
Chapter 18	**What is New in Urticaria? Pathophysiology** M Sendhil Kumaran, Vignesh Narayan	94
	What is New in Urticaria? Diagnosis and Treatment Guillet Carole, Leu Noemi, Schmid-Grendelmeier Peter	98
Chapter 19	**Patient Education Material** Hermenio Lima, Iman Hamed Nasr, Naoko Inomata	103
Chapter 20	**Urticaria in Elderly** Hassan Mobayed, Nasseer Masoodi, Maryam Al-Nesf	110
Chapter 21	**Urticaria in Pregnancy and Lactation** Emek Kocatürk	114
Chapter 22	**Urticaria in Kidney Disease, Liver Disease, and Cardiac Disease** Carla Ritchie	120
Index		123

CHAPTER 1

Urticaria: Introduction and Classification

Jonathan A Bernstein, Michael P Makris,
Germán Darío Ramón

INTRODUCTION

Chronic urticaria (CU) with or without angioedema affects about 1% of the world population and is associated with significant health care and economic burden as well as tremendous impact on health related quality of life. The European Academy of Allergology and Clinical Immunology/Global Allergy and Asthma European Network/European Dermatology Forum/World Allergy Organization (EAACI/GA²LEN/EDF/WAO) guidelines for the definition, classification, diagnosis, and management of urticaria are being updated almost every 4 years; the most recent are published in 2018.[1]

Urticaria is characterized by a central swelling of variable size surrounded by erythema, associated with itching or on occasion a burning sensation that is evanescent with lesions appearing and resolving within 30 minutes to 24 hours.[1] Up to 40% of patients with urticaria may have associated angioedema. Like urticaria, angioedema can appear suddenly involving the lower dermis, subcutis, or mucus membranes but is often more painful than itchy and resolves slower than urticaria over 1–3 days.[1]

CLASSIFICATION

Urticaria is considered acute if present ≤6 weeks and chronic if present >6 weeks.[1] The likelihood of identifying an underlying cause is approximately 15% for acute urticaria and <5% for CU. As urticaria lesions are evanescent, meaning they appear suddenly and disappear typically in <24 hours, the terminology chronic spontaneous urticaria (CSU) has been adapted.[1] Up to 30% of CU sufferers present with the typical skin lesions after certain inducible triggers such as scratching or temperature changes (dermatographism, cold, heat, pressure, sunlight, exercise…); these subsets of CU are called chronic inducible urticarias (CIndUs), substituting the well-known term physical urticaria that was widely used before.[1] These forms of CU can be elicited by specific provocation techniques that will be further discussed in another section.

Table 1 summarizes the classification of CU. Chronic spontaneous urticaria has been further classified based on the presence or absence of specific futures of autoallergy or autoimmunity.[2] It has been shown that the majority of immunoglobulin E (IgE) in CSU patients is autoallergic IgE that in many subjects recognize a

TABLE 1: Classification of chronic urticaria.[1]	
Chronic urticaria subtypes	
Chronic spontaneous urticaria (CSU)	**Chronic inducible urticaria (CIndU)**
Spontaneous appearance of wheals, angioedema, or both for >6 weeks due to known or unknown causes	Symptomatic dermatographism
	Cold urticaria
	Delayed pressure urticaria
	Solar urticaria
	Heat urticaria
	Vibratory urticaria
	Cholinergic urticaria
	Contact urticaria
	Aquagenic urticaria

completely different set of autoantigens than the IgE of healthy individuals; thus type I autoallergy is the main underlying mechanism in this subgroup.[3] On the other hand, patients with IgG autoantibodies to FcεRIα/IgE diagnosed by either positive: Autologous serum skin test (ASST), basophil histamine release assay (BHRA), and/or basophil activation test (BAT) have been classified as having type 2b autoimmunity.[2] It has been recently reported that CSU patients with evidence of autoantibodies such as antinuclear antibodies and/or IgG antithyroid antibodies are more likely to have an associated type 2b autoimmunity, which is important to note clinically as these patients have been found to respond poorly to omalizumab treatment.[2] Other markers that may predict a poor response to omalizumab include a low total IgE and low peripheral blood eosinophil count.[4] Furthermore, a low basophil count has been reported to be associated with a positive basophil activation test and a poor response to omalizumab.[4] In addition, a high D-dimer and also C-reactive protein have been reported to be strong predictors of poor response to second-generation antihistamines, and a positive basophil activation test and possibly a low total IgE are good predictors of response to cyclosporine.[4]

Finally, CSU can be classified histologically by the presence of perivascular lymphocytes with various degrees of mixed infiltrates consisting of eosinophils and/or neutrophils. This differentiation is important as patients with predominantly neutrophilic infiltrates may respond more favorably to certain medications such as dapsone or colchicine.[5]

As more is learned more about the immunopathogenesis for CSU resulting in the discovery of new biomarkers that correlate with patient-specific clinical characteristics and response to therapy, it is predicted that the classification schema for this condition will continue to evolve.[6]

 ONLINE REFERENCES

To access the references of this chapter online, kindly refer to **emedicine360.com** also please follow the instructions mentioned on inside cover.

CHAPTER 2

Etiopathogenesis

Leonor Esteves Caldeira, Célia Costa, Mona Al-Ahmad,
Jorge Sanchez, Ricardo Cardona

INTRODUCTION

Urticaria is a mast cell-driven disease.[1] There are several potential causes of new onset urticaria, although in many patients no specific etiology can be identified. Acute urticaria usually occurs due to exposure to various triggers present in the environment (food, drugs, and insect venom), while in chronic urticaria (CU) these triggers are not usually present, making it more difficult to identify the cause. Different etiologies can activate mast cells through many different mechanisms, which are described hereafter.[2]

MEDIATORS IN THE FORMATION OF THE WHEAL AND ITCHING

Skin mast cell activation is a complex process initiated by diverse stimuli and resulting in three principal effects, namely degranulation, cytokines, and chemokine synthesis and leukotrienes and prostaglandin production.[2,3] The enhanced vascular permeability that results from the release of preformed mediators from mast cells and their delayed generation of cytokines is responsible for the physical manifestation of urticaria.[2]

During degranulation, mast cells release histamine and other inflammatory mediators (e.g., prostaglandins, leukotrienes, cytokines, and chemokines) on activation, which are capable of inducing vasodilation, alteration in endothelial-permeability, plasma extravasation, dermal sensory nerve stimulation, and cell recruitment.[3] Local vasodilatation with increased capillary permeability and plasma leakage results in elevated erythematous wheals. Stimulation of sensory skin nerves contributes along with other mechanisms in skin pruritus and erythematous halo (axon reflex).[4,5] Histamine is a central mediator, as suggested by the prominent clinical symptom of pruritus and the beneficial response to H_1-antihistamines in most of the patients (40–70%). Activation of H_1 receptors in the skin induces itching, flaring, erythema, and wheal, whereas activation of H_2 receptors offer a moderate contribution to erythema and wheal.[6]

Within a 24-hour period after mast cell stimulation cytokines and chemokines are produced. Acute phase cytokines [interleukin (IL)-1 and tumor necrosis factor alpha (TNF-α)] activate the endothelium, allowing recruitment of leukocytes and cytokines synthesis by other cell types, contributing to the maintenance of skin inflammation. Moreover, mast cells can behave as antigen-presenting cells able to activate T-cells and it has been suggested that, by infiltrating the skin, T-cells participate in the chronicity of the lesions. This could explain why some patients with H_1 antagonist-resistant CU can be improved by immunosuppressants that target T-cells, such as cyclosporine.[7]

Leukotrienes and prostaglandins are produced from arachidonic acid in the hours following mast cell activation. Two enzymatic systems, cyclo-oxygenases and lipoxygenases, participate in this production. Leukotriene synthesis is thought to happen in the early and selective recruitment of leukocytes, but the mechanisms by which they participate in the urticarial lesions are not established. Similarly with cytokines, these mediators are thought to be important for the chronicity of the disease.[8]

MAST CELL ACTIVATION MECHANISMS IN URTICARIA

The mast cell has >36 membrane receptors that can generate its activation and release from the preformed granules (**Fig. 1**). These receptors can be activated by immunological mechanisms (innate or adaptive response) or by nonimmunological mechanisms.[2] Although many of these mechanisms can overlap and are not mutually exclusive, we will present them separately for academic purposes. Among the immunological mechanisms, the adaptive response has been the most studied.

Immunoglobulin E (IgE)-mediated urticaria [type I hypersensitivity (HS)]: This immediate HS mechanism is present in acute urticaria and is initiated by antigen-mediated IgE immune complexes that bind and cross-link Fc receptors on the surface of mucosa/skin mast cells and blood basophils, which became activated and degranulate. Common allergens that can result in acute urticaria include foods, food additives, and drugs (particularly antibiotics and painkillers). The most common foods associated with the condition in children are milk, eggs, peanuts, tree nuts, and soybeans. In adults, fish, shellfish, tree nuts, and peanuts are most often implicated. Beta-lactams, namely penicillins and cephalosporins, are the

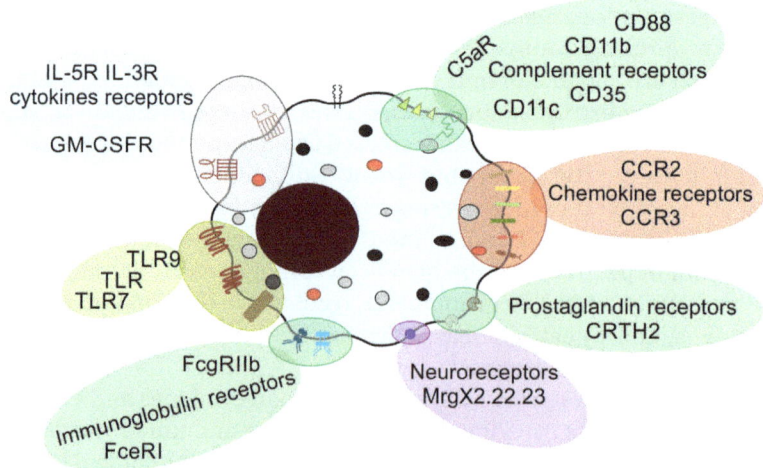

FIG. 1: Mast cell receptors involved in the pathogenesis of urticaria.

antibiotics most implicated in causing urticaria by this immediate HS mechanism. Insect stings may also be associated with acute urticaria and, in some cases, to anaphylaxis. The stinging insects that frequently cause severe allergic reactions include bees, vespids, and fire ants. Acute urticaria may also occur in latex allergy, after contact with latex-containing products, including latex gloves and balloons.[8] In CU, these exogenous triggers are not usually the cause of the disease but can occasionally cause exacerbations as is the case with nonsteroidal anti-inflammatory drugs (NSAIDs).[9-11]

Patients with chronic spontaneous urticaria (CSU) have a higher total IgE concentration and also a higher frequency of atopy.[12-15] In addition, IgE autoantibodies to thyroid autoantigens such as thyroperoxidase (TPO) and thyroglobulin are present in 15–40% of CSU patients.[16-19] What has been described as an "autoallergic" reaction.[20,21] Why these autoantibodies are formed is unknown, but some mechanisms have been proposed like molecular mimicry with some environmental antigens or molecular spreading as a consequence of chronic inflammation. Several in vitro studies show that IgE antibodies against TPO, tissue factor, IL24, can induce the activation of mast cells and basophils.[18,22-24] Also a recent study[19] demonstrated that the inoculation of TPO into the skin of patients with CSU and anti-TPO IgE can induce the formation of hives in the skin; additionally, this reaction could be reproduced in healthy subjects with passive transfer of serum with anti-TPO IgE at the subcutaneous level.

IgG-mediated urticaria (type II HS): A subpopulation of patients with CU has been referred to have an autoimmune etiology (40-45%) in which there is IgG antibodies against to the α-subunit of the high-affinity IgE receptor (FcεRIα) (35–40%) or to IgE itself (IgG anti-IgE; 5–10%). The presence of IgM against these autoantigens has also been detected but less frequently (**Fig. 2**). These autoantibodies can be

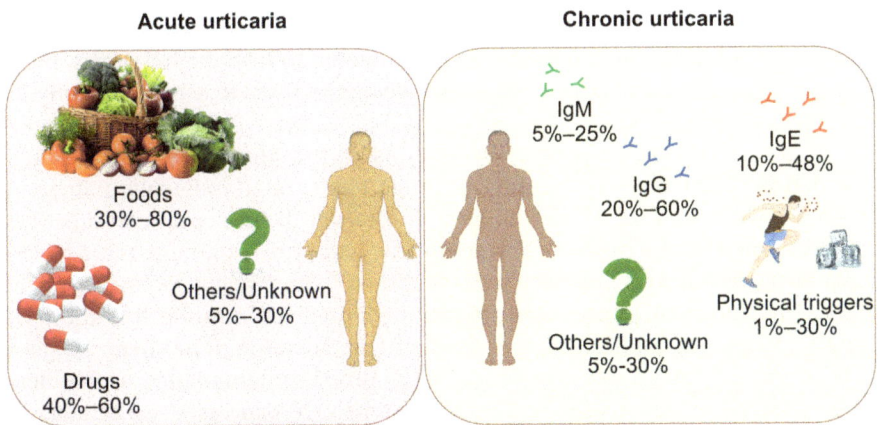

FIG. 2: Mechanisms and triggers of acute and chronic urticaria: The frequency described is wide since it varies according to the age group and study reports. In acute urticaria, food and drugs are the main triggers and can induce the disease through IgE mechanisms, enzymatic reaction or by irritative effects that induce degranulation of mast cells. In CU, several autoantigens detected by IgE, IgG, and IgM can induce the disease, however, there seem to be other mechanisms that have not been described, such as those of urticarias induced by physical stimuli like ice or exercise.

demonstrated by basophil histamine release assay or by autologous serum skin testing. For activation to occur it is necessary cross-linking IgE receptors or adjacent IgE molecules by these antibodies. Histamine release is augmented by complement activation with release of C5a. As a group, symptoms are more severe and last longer in this subpopulation of patients than in patients without such autoantibodies. Associated autoimmune phenomena include a higher incidence of antithyroid antibodies, which may result in Hashimoto thyroiditis, as well as positive antinuclear antibodies.[11,19,25,26]

Beyond the autoimmune mechanisms, other mechanisms have been described as related to the pathogenesis of CU, involves dysregulation of intracellular signaling pathways within mast cells and basophils that lead to defects in trafficking or function of these cells, as it will be explained below.

Circulating immune complex (CIC)-mediated urticaria (type III HS): There is a paucity of literature describing the role of CIC in urticaria. Nevertheless, it is known that antigen-antibody complex interacts with receptors for the Fc portion of Igs (FcR) on several cell types, including mast cells and basophils. This mechanism is possibly responsible for the urticarial flares observed in the course of infectious diseases and lupus erythematosus, in which high quantities of CIC are produced.[27]

On the other hand, nonimmunological urticarias are the urticarias which are not mediated by effectors of adaptive immunity. Mast cells express a number of surface receptors, which, upon binding to various molecules, are able to initiate a signal to trigger degranulation, specifically, receptors for neurotransmitters, neurohormones, and neuropeptides; toll-like receptors; receptors for the complement molecules and cytokine and chemokine receptors.[28]

Emotional and psychological factors, such as depression, anxiety, and stress, seems to play a contributory role in the onset of the disease and in its evolution. Additionally, emotional stress contributes to flare-ups of urticaria, which might be explained by the activation pathways transduced by receptors for neurotransmitters, neurohormones, and neuropeptides, particularly substance P.[4] It is worth mentioning that, patients with CSU seem to have higher cortisol levels than healthy controls and their basophils have been shown to active promptly with stress-related neuropeptides.[29]

It is not clear how infection contributes to the genesis, perpetuation, or exacerbation of CU. Notwithstanding, pathogen-associated molecular patterns on microbes have been found to be able to bind to toll-like receptors on mast cells, causing degranulation. The most frequently involved type of pathogens are bacteria and viruses, often linked to acute viral infections.[30] Other proposed mechanism of urticaria development, as previously mentioned, involves immune activation, with immune complex formation and/or complement activation. It has been suggested that infection may play a role in the onset of CSU and its maintenance, and cofactors like stress may be necessary for the CSU phenotype to be expressed, especially when urticaria develops in context of severe infections like pneumonia or pyelonephritis. On the other hand, some patients improve by the discovery and treatment of occult infections.[29] The infectious agents commonly associated with urticaria include various viruses (e.g., rhinovirus, rotavirus, Epstein–Barr, hepatitis A, hepatitis B, hepatitis C, herpes simplex, and human immunodeficiency virus), bacteria (e.g., urinary tract infections, dental infections, *Helicobacter pylori*, and *Mycoplasma pneumonia*), and parasites (e.g., *Ancylostoma, Strongyloides, Schistosoma mansoni, Anisakis simplex,* and *Blastocystis hominis*).[8]

Complements, such as C5a anaphylatoxin, can also trigger mast cell degranulation by binding to their respective receptors available on mast cell surface, independent of the involvement of IgE or IgE receptors.[31]

In what concerns chronic inducible urticarias (CIndU) they probably result from heightened sensitivity by the mast cell to environmental conditions, although the exact pathogenesis is too unknown.[1] As many patients document the efficacy of anti-IgE (omalizumab), a possible role of IgE in the degranulation of mast cells in CIndU has been suggested. Type I autoimmunity, is defended in several studies to be of major importance in the pathogenesis of CIndU. It is thought that environmental stimuli induce a neoantigen, specific to IgE antibody that binds to mast cells. In support of this, it has been described that in symptomatic dermographism, cold and solar urticaria, the disease is passively transferable by transfer of serum, being IgE the suggested transferable serum factor. Also, in solar urticaria, specific photo-induced autoantigens have been documented to bind to IgE on mast cells and in cold urticaria desensitization was shown after depletion of a cold-dependent skin antigen that could activate mast cells.[32,33] In cholinergic urticaria, specific IgE antibodies to autologous sweat antigens or skin resident fungi, *Malassezia globosa*, have been reported.[4] On the other hand, and as already mentioned, mast cells and basophils may also be activated through IgE-independent pathways. Recently, in physical urticaria, it has been being investigated if there is any participation of transient receptor potential (TRP) channels which can be regulated by changes in temperature, pH, or osmolality and produce calcium influx into the cells. However, its role in CIndU is still unknown.[32]

SUMMARY AND CLINICAL APPLICATION OF THIS KNOWLEDGE

The recent description of anti-IL24 IgE in 90–100% of patients with CSU compared to only 10% of subjects without urticaria, opens the door to the use of these autoantibodies as a confirmatory diagnostic test.[34] The presence or not of IgE anti-TPO and IgG anti-IgE among other autoantibodies seems to define different endophenotypes of patients[25] (**Table 1**); those with IgE anti-TPO are more frequently associated with a reaction with NSAIDs, a better response with omalizumab and the presence of rhinitis or asthma. In contrast, those with IgG autoantibodies are more frequently associated with the presence of inducible urticaria in addition to CSU, a better response with cyclosporine, and a lower response with antihistamines. Therefore, these biomarkers have the potential to transform the clinical approach in CSU at the level of diagnosis, treatment, and prognosis.

TABLE 1: Each cross represents the frequency of the diseases found in previous studies.

	IgE autoantibodies	IgG autoantibodies
Asthma	+++	+
Atopy	+++	+
Total IgE	++	+
NSAIDs reactions	+++	+
Inducible urticaria and CSU together	++	+++
Autoimmune diseases	+	+*
Cyclosporine response	+++	+++**
Omalizumab response	+++***	+++

+: <25% of the patients, ++: 25–50%, and +++: >51%.

* Although the frequency of autoimmune diseases seems to be <25% in both groups, some studies suggest a predominance of their presence in patients with IgG autoantibodies.
**Some studies suggest that it is better in patients with IgG autoantibodies.
***Some studies suggest that it is better in patients with IgE autoantibodies.

(CSU: chronic spontaneous urticaria; IgG: immunoglobulin G; NSAIDs: nonsteroidal anti-inflammatory drugs)

 ONLINE REFERENCES

To access the references of this chapter online, kindly refer to **emedicine360.com** also please follow the instructions mentioned on inside cover.

CHAPTER 3

Acute Urticaria

Kanokvalai Kulthanan, Angèle Soria, Iris Medina

DEFINITION

Acute urticaria (AU) is defined as the occurrence of spontaneous wheals, angioedema or both that has been evolving for <6 weeks,[1] with flare-ups lasting a few hours, which may recur on several consecutive days. Although AU is most often nonallergic, it is important not to ignore an allergic cause. In extreme cases of allergy, patients may develop anaphylactic shock.

EPIDEMIOLOGY

Approximately 12–23.5% of the population will experience AU at some time in their life.[2,3] The prevalence of AU is higher in individuals with atopic diseases.[3]

CLINICAL ASPECTS

The disease is characterized by the sudden appearance of wheals which is a cutaneous swelling of variable sizes, invariably surrounded by a reflex erythema, with associated itching or, sometimes, a burning sensation. Wheals are transient with the skin returning to its normal appearance in usually 1–24 hours (**Fig. 1**).

In some patients, wheals are accompanied by angioedema, or only angioedema is present.

Angioedema is characterized by a sudden and pronounced swelling of the deep dermis and subcutaneous tissue or mucous membranes, with a painful rather than an itching sensation. Angioedema has a slower resolution than wheals that can take up to 72 hours (**Fig. 2**).

Some patients may have systemic symptoms such as shortness of breath, dyspnea, dizziness, headache, nausea, diarrhea, abdominal pain or even anaphylaxis. Patients with extensive wheals tended to have co-existing angioedema and also a statistically significant higher percentage of systemic symptoms.[4]

Acute Nonallergic Urticaria

Various factors or triggers favor its appearance in a predisposed terrain (**Box 1**).

Infections

Numerous infections, particularly viral, may be preceded or accompanied by AU, especially in children. The reported prevalence of upper respiratory tract infections

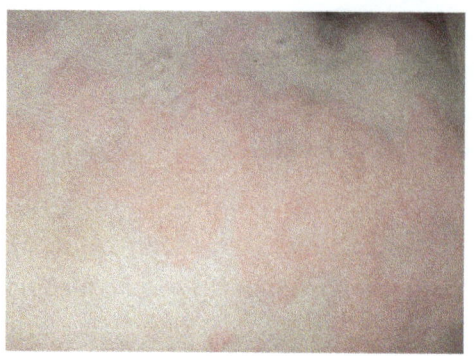

FIG. 1: Urticaria wheals.

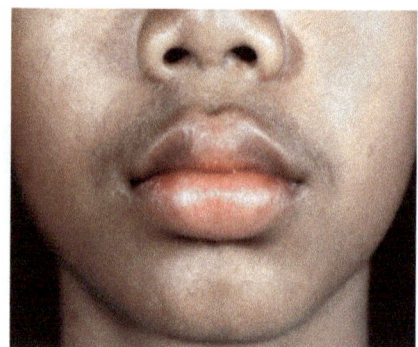

FIG. 2: Angioedema of lips.

> **Box 1: Acute urticaria and triggers.**
>
> - Infections
>   - Viral
>   - Bacterial
>   - Parasitic
> - Medications
>   - Nonsteroidal anti-inflammatory drugs
>   - Antibiotics
>   - Radiocontrast media
> - Foods
> - Insect stings
>   - Bees
>   - Fire ants
>   - Hornets
>   - Wasps
>   - Yellow jackets
> - Contact allergy
> - Blood transfusions
> - Vaccinations
> - No triggering factor

in AU ranged from 28 to 62%.[4,5] Infections can occur before, during or shortly after onset of urticaria.[6] The example of viral agents includes cytomegalovirus, coxsackie A9 virus, hepatitis A, hepatitis B virus, herpes simplex virus, parvovirus B19, and Epstein–Barr virus. Other reported infectious agents include *Mycoplasma pneumoniae, Strongyloides stercoralis, Plasmodium falciparum, Anisakis simplex,* etc.[7-14] Urticaria eruptions associated with Coronavirus disease 2019 (COVID-19) have been recently reported.[15] Urticarial lesions associated with fever were reported to be early or even prodromal signs of COVID-19, in the absence of respiratory symptoms.[16]

However, it is sometimes difficult to say whether AU is due to the virus and/or secondary to the drugs prescribed for this infectious episode.

Drugs

Drugs can elicit AU both as immunoglobulin E (IgE)-mediated with immediate hypersensitivity reaction with risk of severe anaphylaxis, or nonallergic hypersensitivity reactions for example with inhibitors of cyclo-oxygenase drugs as aspirin or nonsteroidal anti-inflammatory drugs (NSAIDs), but a true immediate hypersensitivity reaction can occur with these drugs too.[17,18] Multiple medications including antibiotics (beta-lactam), NSAIDs, fluoroquinolones or iodinated contrast products are associated with development of urticaria. In this case, there is no risk of anaphylaxis, as these reactions are not mediated by IgE. Vaccines may also be responsible.

Foods

Patients with AU frequently suspect that foods are the causes of their lesions. However, many studies have shown that food allergy such as cow's milk or food intolerance are more frequently implied in children.[19,20] In adult patients, food was not shown to be the causing agent of AU.[4,5]

Others

Other potential causes of AU include insect bites or stings, contact allergy, blood transfusion and vaccination. However, in many cases, it is not exceptional to identify a triggering factor.

Acute Allergic Urticaria

It is the questioning that makes it possible, depending on the context and especially the chronology of events, to evoke an allergic AU. In this case, the chronology is suggestive, with exposition with the allergen occurring in the hour or at most the 2 hours preceding the outbreak of AU. The triggers for such AU are drugs, foods (e.g., sea food, eggs, and colored food), insect venoms (wasps, bees, hornets, and bumblebees), and certain substances in contact with the skin. In the vast majority of cases, AU is accompanied by general signs (palmoplantar pruritus, arterial hypotension, dyspnea, diarrhea, abdominal pain, vomiting, sweating, malaise, and in extreme cases anaphylactic shock).

The severity of the clinical picture should be assessed according to the Ring and Messmer classification. This AU is always of rapid resolution, lasting no >24 hours, with a new exposure to the allergen often leading to a faster and more severe recurrence. In the acute phase, it is recommended to perform a blood test for tryptase, if possible 1 hour 30 minutes to 2 hours after the onset of the manifestations, and later after 24 hours have elapsed, in order to determine the baseline level. An elevated plasma tryptase level within 2 hours of clinical onset indicates anaphylaxis.

Special forms of acute allergic urticaria, occurring >2 hours after allergen exposition and must be known.

Special forms of Acute Allergic Urticaria

- Exercise-induced food anaphylaxis
- Alpha-galactosidase anaphylaxis
- *Anisakis* simplex anaphylaxis
- AU of immunological contact

Diagnostic Workup

In general, AU is usually self-limiting and not evocative to allergic factor, and does not require routine diagnostic tests unless strongly suggested by patient history.[1] Careful history taking and physical examination are very important. Diagnostic workup is indicated only when immediate hypersensitivity; i.e., type I hypersensitivity, is suspected to be the underlying cause.[1] Most IgE mediated hypersensitivity reactions occur rapidly, usually within 2 hours of exposure.

In case of suspected AU allergy, skin tests (prick tests, and intradermal tests) should be performed later approximately 4–6 weeks after the original reaction took place. Pending this assessment, any further exposure to the suspected allergen(s) is forbidden and an emergency kit containing an autoinjectable syringe of adrenaline/epinephrine is prescribed.

Treatment[1]

Avoidance of Trigger if Identified

The first-line treatment of AU is second generation H_1-antihistamines, which may be increased up to four times the standard dosage until there is a resolution. The new generation of nonsedating H_1-antihistamines are effective rapidly.

The second-line of treatment is a short course of corticosteroids, adding on nonsedating H_1-antihistamine.

In severe cases or anaphylaxis, medications include epinephrine, inhaled beta 2-agonists for bronchospasm, antihistamines, vasopressors, and corticosteroids.[21] Prednisolone 0.5 mg/kg can be given for 5–10 days. Only first generation H_1-antihistamines are available for parenteral use.

Acute Urticaria without Signs of Severity

- Eviction of the triggering factor(s)
- Prescription of a second generation H_1-antihistamines at the usual dosage for a few days. This is a practice consensus, as no study has compared H_1-antihistamines with placebo.

Acute Urticaria with Manifestations of Anaphylaxis or Suspected Anaphylaxis

Management depends on the severity of the manifestations. In all cases, the patient should be placed in the Trendelenburg position. The first line of treatment in case of anaphylactic shock is adrenaline (epinephrine). Other treatment depends on the symptoms and include oxygen therapy, vascular filling, bronchodilator if bronchospasm, and H_1-antihistamines. Corticosteroids are of limited value in the treatment of the acute phase, given their long duration of action. Any patient who has had an anaphylactic incident should have an allergological consultation. An emergency kit containing self-injectable adrenaline/epinephrine should be prescribed, with education of the patient and his or her family.

Natural Course

The prognosis of AU is excellent, with most cases resolving within days. Up to 56–70% of the patients with AU had complete remissions within 1 week, 78.5–86%, within 2 weeks, and 91–96%, within 3 weeks.[4-17] Up to 25% of cases present with AU were reported to turn out to have chronic urticaria.[4,22]

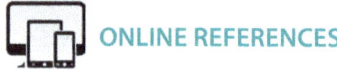 ONLINE REFERENCES

To access the references of this chapter online, kindly refer to **emedicine360.com** also please follow the instructions mentioned on inside cover.

CHAPTER 4

Chronic Spontaneous Urticaria

Kiran V Godse, Abhishek De

INTRODUCTION

Urticaria is a condition characterized by the development of wheals (hives), angioedema, or both. A wheal is a specific skin lesion for urticaria that has a central swelling of variable size and surrounded by a zone of reflex erythema; it is usually associated with an itching and is of a fleeting nature lasting <24 hours. Angioedema on the other hand is characterized by a sudden, pronounced erythematous or skin-colored swelling of the lower dermis and subcutis or mucous membranes; is usually associated with pain, rather than itch and its resolution is slower than that of wheals (can take up to 72 hours). Majority of patients present with isolated hives; about one-third of patients present with both hives and angioedema.[1]

Urticaria can be classified according to duration and etiology, although more than two types of urticaria can coexist in the same patient. Chronic urticaria (CU) is defined as urticaria present daily or almost daily for 6 weeks or more. CU can be further classified into chronic inducible urticaria (CINDU), and chronic spontaneous urticaria (CSU). In this chapter, we will mostly deal with CSU.[1]

EPIDEMIOLOGY

Lifetime prevalence for any type of urticaria range from <1 to 24%, whereas, the overall point prevalence of CSU across all age groups is estimated at 0.7%, which may vary from 0.23 to 1.8% in different geographic locations. Recent data suggests there is an increase in point prevalence over time.[2]

The prevalence of CSU is high in all age groups, highest among those 40–60 years of age. CSU is equally common in children as it is in adults estimated on average at 1%.

There is a strong female predilection, affecting women twice as often as men (1.3% vs. 0.8%). This difference is less evident in the elderly, children, and for cholinergic urticaria and delayed pressure urticaria (DPU). Sex differences are absent in children, a point prevalence of 1.0% for girls and 1.1% for boys.[3]

PATHOGENESIS

It is important to know the recent understanding of the cellular and molecular pathogenesis of CSU, to realize the potential therapeutic targets.

Cellular Components of Chronic Spontaneous Urticaria

Mast cells and basophils are the most important inflammatory cells involved in the pathogenesis of urticaria.

Mast Cells

Cutaneous mast cells degranulation releases inflammatory mediators such as histamine, proteases, and cytokines along with the generation of platelet-activating factor and arachidonic acid metabolites like prostaglandin D2 (PGD2) and leukotrienes C4, D4, and E4; which essentially leads to the characteristic symptoms of CSU such as wheal, angioedema, and pruritus.

Mast cells have two types namely MCT and MCTC. MCT type of mast cells are tryptase-positive, chymase-negative, and T-lymphocyte dependent cells found mainly in the mucosal tissues. On the other hand MCTC are both tryptase-positive and chymase-positive, and T-lymphocyte-independent cells which are found mainly in skin and gastrointestinal submucosa. The number of MCTC type of mast cells are much higher in skin tissues obtained from patients with CU than that of healthy controls.[4-7]

Basophils

Basopenia may be associated with active or severe CSU. It is generally believed that the basopenia occurs because of the migration of basophils from blood to skin.

Eosinophils

Eosinopenia may also be associated with CSU. Eosinophils, in combination with mast cells and basophils, possibly have a role in priming the skin for wheal formation.[8]

Lymphocytes

Lesional skin in CSU demonstrates CD4 T lymphocytes infiltrate with minimal B cells. These CD4 lymphocytes demonstrate characteristics of both T-helper 1 (TH1) and T-helper 2 (TH2) cells.[9]

CHRONIC SPONTANEOUS URTICARIA AND AUTOIMMUNITY

The degranulation of cutaneous mast cells causes the development of skin changes, such as sensory nerve stimulation, vasodilation, and extravasation. This process also help in the recruitment of basophils, eosinophils, and T cells. These cellular and molecular changes finally lead to the characteristic symptoms of wheal, pruritus, and angioedema.

Two groups of mast cell-degranulating signals have been identified:
1. Immunoglobulin E (IgE) autoantibodies to autoallergens; and
2. Autoantibodies that target activating mast cell-receptors

On this basis most patients of CSU are caused by two types of autoimmune hypersensitivity, the first one is the type I autoimmunity (autoallergic CSU) and the other one is the type IIb autoimmunity (autoimmune CSU).[10]

In the autoallergic CSU type, autoantigens crosslink IgE autoantibodies on mast cells and basophils to cause the release of vasoactive mediators. Involvement of the type 1 hypersensitivity was identified decades earlier by the association of IgE with

CSU. Most studies suggested IgE autoantibodies are responsible for the increased total IgE levels in CSU patients. Studies have demonstrated thyroperoxidase (TPO) to be a common and relevant autoallergen in CSU. Autoallergic CSU patients also have IgE autoantibodies directed to many autoantigens beyond TPO, which include thyroglobulin, tissue factor, and interleukin-24 (IL-24).[11]

Much later, a type IIb hypersensitivity mechanism was described in CSU which is due to mast cell-targeted IgG or IgM autoantibodies.[11]

Recent understandings of CSU, thus point toward two endotypes of CSU: (1) Type I autoimmunity or autoallergy; and (2) Type IIb autoimmunity (**Table 1** and **Fig. 1**).

FACTORS ASSOCIATED OR AGGRAVATING CHRONIC SPONTANEOUS URTICARIA

Infections

Though infections such as bacterial, viral, parasitic, or fungal have been implicated as etiological factors of CSU, it could never be confirmed as causal association. Some cases of recurrent urticaria in the Mediterranean region had been associated with

TABLE 1: Features of type I and type IIB autoimmune CSU.

Features	Type I autoimmunity or autoallergy	Type IIb autoimmunity
Autoantibodies	Auto-IgE (e.g., against TPO, TG, TF, IL-24, and dsDNA)	Auto-IgG (against IgE and FcεRI)
Diagnosis	Total auto-IgE and specific IgE to autoallergens in type I	Triple positivity: BHRA/BAT + ASST + WB/ELISA + in type IIb
Disease activity/severity	Tends to be lower	Tends to be higher
Disease duration	Tends to be shorter	Tends to be longer
Rates of concomitant autoimmune diseases	Might be higher	Might be lower
Total IgE levels	Normal or high	Low
Basopenia rates	Might be lower	Might be higher
Eosinopenia rates	Tend to be lower	Tend to be higher
C-reactive protein levels	May be lower	May be higher
Responder rates to sgAHs	May be higher	May be lower
Responder rates to omalizumab	Higher	Lower
Speed of response to omalizumab	Faster	Slower
Immunosuppressive therapy	Has less importance	Can be more effective

(ANA: antinuclear antibodies; ASST: autologous serum skin test; WB: Western blot; BHRA: basophil histamine release assay; BAT: basophil activation test; CRP: C-reactive protein; CSU: chronic spontaneous urticaria; dsDNA: double-stranded DNA; ELISA: enzyme-linked immunosorbent assay; IL: interleukin; TPO: thyroperoxidase; TG: thyroglobulin; TF: tissue factor; sgAHs: second-generation antihistamines)

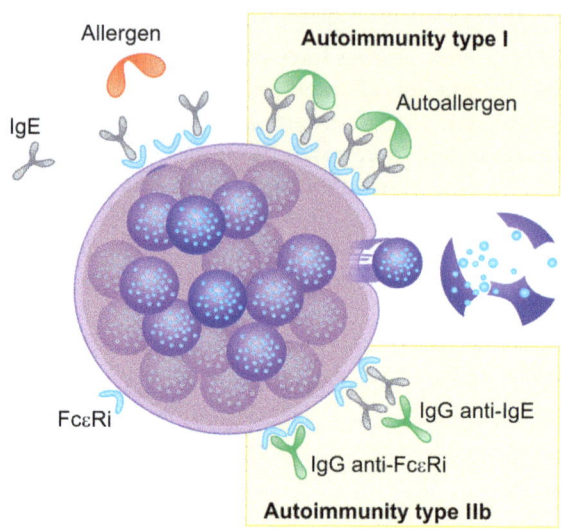

(CSU: chronic spontaneous urticaria; IgE: immunoglobulin E)

FIG. 1: Endotypes of CSU.

Anisakis simplex, a sea fish nematode. *Helicobacter pylori* was also often implicated in CSU, but there are conflicting evidences for this association.[12]

Food

True type I food allergy must be a rare cause of CSU, though patients often associate foods and food additives with symptom onset. Studies have shown <30% resolution 10–14 days after removal of pseudoallergens from patients' diets.[12]

Drugs

Angiotensin-converting enzyme (ACE) inhibitors and nonsteroidal anti-inflammatory drugs (NSAIDs) are most commonly implicated as the causes of urticaria.[12]

Emotional Stress

Patients with CSU experience high rates of anxiety, depression, and somatoform disorders; but it is uncertain if emotional stress/anxiety is the cause or consequence of CSU.[12]

Clinical Manifestations

The characteristic symptoms of CSU are wheals with or without angioedema. Individual wheal lesions usually last <24 hours, although new wheals keep occurring in different areas.

Angioedema is defined as a sudden, ill-defined swelling in subcutaneous, or submucosal tissue. Angioedema last longer than hives for about 48–72 hours. Most common sites for angioedema are lip, tongue, eyelids, genitalia, and bowel. CSU is associated with angioedema in 40% of patients.

Urticaria may occur at any time, but many report the worst episodes are usually in the evening or night and may cause sleep disturbances. CSU causes substantial impairment in quality-of-life, including self-image, sexual relationships, and social interaction. Women may have premenstrual exacerbations. Severe CSU attacks may be associated with systemic symptoms of fatigue, lassitude, sweats and chills, indigestion, or arthralgias.[13]

CHRONIC SPONTANEOUS URTICARIA AND ASSOCIATION OF OTHER DISEASES

Chronic urticaria has been associated with various autoimmune diseases including autoimmune thyroid diseases, vitiligo, insulin-dependent diabetes, rheumatoid arthritis, and pernicious anemia. A possible association between *H. pylori* gastritis and CU was suggested by some studies. Among women, CSU was found to be significantly associated with atopic dermatitis, allergic rhinitis, autoimmune thyroid diseases, systemic lupus, vitiligo, and Henoch–Schönlein purpura. Among men, CSU was significantly associated with atopic dermatitis, allergic rhinitis, autoimmune thyroid diseases, Kawasaki disease, and inflammatory bowel disease.[14]

Almost one out of three CSU patients has at least one underlying psychiatric disorder. Depression and anxiety symptoms were found to be more common in patients with CSU than in the control group.[15]

Chronic viral infections including those by hepatitis B virus and hepatitis C virus have been reported to be comorbidities of CSU. However, recent meta-analysis suggested hepatitis B/C infections are unlikely to be linked to CSU.[16] In urticaria-patients, the prevalence of gastroesophageal reflux disease (GERD) was four-fold higher than in control without hives.[17]

Natural History

There is no evidence that the natural history of CSU is influenced by treatment. An earlier review of authors who have reported a course for CSU, where 50% of all cases will resolve (with or without treatment) within 6 months of onset, and 2% may persist for 25 years (**Fig. 2**).

However, recent studies suggested that the median duration of CSU can be of 4 years and about one-third of patients having a relapsing/remitting course.

Longer median duration of disease is seen in the patients with a more relapsing course, and in patients with angioedema. Younger age of presentation compared to older age tends to have a longer course of disease.[18]

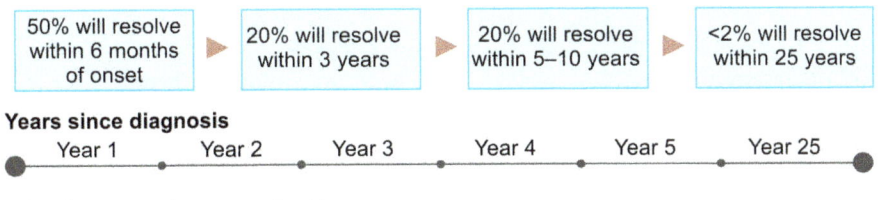

(CSU: chronic spontaneous urticaria)

FIG. 2: Suggested natural course of CSU.

DIAGNOSIS

Diagnosis of urticaria is mostly clinical. The diagnostic workup of CSU should target to (i) exclude other differential diagnoses (**Box 1**) (ii) assess disease activity, impact, and control, and (iii) identify triggers of exacerbation or, where indicated, any underlying causes.

International guidelines suggest detailed history with pertinent questions to be taken (**Box 2**). Thorough physical examination of the patient is of extreme importance.

In a patient of CSU the recommended tests are complete blood count with five part differentials including absolute basophil count and absolute eosinophil counts, erythrocyte sedimentation rate, and/or C-reactive protein, IgE, and thyroid hormones and autoantibodies.

It is advisable to avoid too many tests in CSU, but if indicated by history and/or physical examination, like in cases where individual lesions are lasting for >24 hours, hives are associated with purpura or tenderness, or there is presence of systemic symptoms; a skin biopsy specimen may be required to rule out vasculitis.

In selected patients, more extended investigations including ruling out infectious diseases such as *H. pylori*, performing allergy skin tests, and/or allergen avoidance tests; may be required.

Currently, the only available tests to screen for autoantibodies against either IgE or FcεR1 are the autologous serum skin test (ASST) and basophil activation tests (BATs).[12,13]

Patient-reported Outcome Measures in Chronic Spontaneous Urticaria

Different patient-reported outcome measures (PROMs) such as the urticaria activity score (UAS), the CU quality of life questionnaire (CU-Q2oL), and the urticaria control test (UCT) are suggested to be used in clinical practice and research to delineate the impact of CSU on patients and the impact of treatment on disease control, keep the patient engaged in the management and assist as a research tool. Of these tools some can only be used prospectively (e.g., UAS) and others, can be used retrospectively (e.g., UCT). Patients should be assessed with PROMs at the first and then every follow-up visit.[19]

Box 1: Differential diagnosis of chronic spontaneous urticaria (CSU).

- Urticarial vasculitis
- Erythema multiforme
- Figurate erythemas
- Toxic erythema
- Bullous pemphigoid—prodromal lesions
- Erysipelas
- Cellulitis
- Systemic lupus erythematosus
- Progesterone-induced dermatosis
- Hansen disease

> **Box 2: Recommended questions to be involved in history taking in chronic spontaneous urticaria (CSU).**
>
> - Time of onset of disease
> - Frequency/Duration of and provoking factors for wheals
> - Diurnal variation
> - Occurrence in relation to weekends, holidays, and foreign travel
> - Shape, size, and distribution of wheals
> - Associated angioedema
> - Associated subjective symptoms of lesions, e.g., pruritus and pain
> - Family and personal history regarding urticaria or atopy
> - Previous or current allergies, infections, internal diseases, or other possible causes
> - Psychosomatic and psychiatric diseases
> - Surgical implantations and events during surgery, e.g., after local anesthesia
> - Gastric/Intestinal problems
> - Induction by physical agents or exercise
> - Use of drugs (i.e., nonsteroidal anti-inflammatory drugs, immunizations, hormones, laxatives, ear and eye drops, and alternative remedies)
> - Observed correlation to food
> - Relationship to the menstrual cycle
> - Smoking habits (especially use of perfumed tobacco products or cannabis)
> - Type of work
> - Hobbies
> - Stress
> - Quality of life-related to urticaria and emotional impact

MANAGEMENT

The aim of CSU management should be to treat the disease effectively and safely until it is gone. The therapeutic approach to CSU should include: (1) identification and elimination of underlying causes, (2) the avoidance of eliciting factors, (3) the use of pharmacological treatment for complete symptom control as much as possible the safety and the quality of life of each individual patient.

General Management

- Patients with CSU should discontinue medication that is suspected to worsen the disease, for example, NSAIDs.
- Chronic spontaneous urticaria is rarely reported to be associated with inflammatory diseases like reflux esophagitis or infectious diseases, such as *H. pylori* infection, bacterial infections of the nasopharynx, or bowel parasites. It is not easily possible to discern whether any of these are relevant causes of CSU but these conditions should be treated appropriately.
- Immunoglobulin E-mediated food allergy or non-IgE-mediated hypersensitivity reactions (pseudoallergic reactions) to food ingredients or food additives were

identified extremely rarely as the underlying cause of CSU. If identified, the specific food allergens need to be omitted as far as possible.

First Line of Pharmacological Management

- Second-generation H_1-antihistamines are recommended as first-line treatment of CSU by most guidelines. Second-generation antihistamines are minimally or nonsedating and free of anticholinergic effects.
- It is recommended that second-generation H_1-antihistamines be taken regularly for the treatment of patients with CSU and not as and when required.
- Nonsedating second-generation H_1-antihistamines which have extensive efficacy and safety data available, are cetirizine, desloratadine, fexofenadine, levocetirizine, loratadine, ebastine, rupatadine, and bilastine.
- Older first-generation H_1-antihistamines are not preferred in the management of CSU as they have pronounced anticholinergic and sedative effects and have many interactions with alcohol and drugs.
- In the management of CSU, one should aim for complete symptom control.[1]

Second Line of Pharmacological Management

- Patient, no responding to standard pharmacological doses, second-generation H_1-antihistamines can be up-dosed up to 4-fold.
- Researches suggest that, most patients with CSU, who are initially not responding to standard pharmacological doses, do benefit from up-dosing of H_1-antihistamines.[1]
- A recent meta-analysis suggested that the rate of response to H_1-antihistamines improves from 38.6% in standard doses to 63.2% when up dosed to 4-fold.
- In general, use of different H_1-antihistamines at the same time is not recommended.[10]

Third Line of Pharmacological Management

Omalizumab

- The European Academy of Allergology and Clinical Immunology/Global Allergy and Asthma European Network/European Dermatology Forum/World Allergy Organization (EAACI/GA2LEN/EDF/WAO) guideline suggest the use of omalizumab for patients unresponsive to 4-fold up dosed second-generation H_1-antagonists.[1]
- Omalizumab is a humanized monoclonal IgG antibody against IgE, with low immunogenicity and is the only nonantihistamine drug licensed for the treatment of CSU.
- Omalizumab binds to free IgE, which reduces free IgE levels. It also down-regulates FcεRI receptors on basophils and mast cell.
- Omalizumab works in CSU by:
  - Reducing the release ability of mast cells
  - Improving basophil count and basophil IgE-receptor function
  - Decreasing the action of IgG autoantibodies against FcεRI and IgE
  - Decreasing the action of IgE autoantibodies against antigens or autoantigens which may be the driving factors for CSU (hitherto unidentified)
- Randomized controlled trials (RCTs) suggest a 71% of reduction of itch is noted with omalizumab at the end of 12 weeks of treatment. 44% of the patients may achieve a UAS7 score of zero at the end of 3 months of treatment.

- In CSU, omalizumab prevents angioedema development, improves quality of life, is suitable for long-term treatment, and effectively treats relapse after discontinuation.
- The recommended dose of omalizumab in CSU is 300 mg every 4 weeks. Dosing is independent of total serum IgE.[20]

Fourth Line of Pharmacological Management

Cyclosporine
- The most effective of the remaining options at present is cyclosporine; supported by double-blind RCTs.
- The EAACI/GA2LEN/EDF/WAO guideline recommends the use of cyclosporine A for the patients with CSU unresponsive to second generation H_1-antihistamines and omalizumab.[1]
- Indian consensus for the management of urticaria recommends cyclosporine A as a third line of treatment for CSU not responding to up-dosed second generation H_1-antihistamines along with omalizumab.[21]
- Though cyclosporine A has a higher incidence of adverse effects; it has a much better risk/benefit ratio in comparison to long-term use of steroids.
- Cyclosporine A is an off-label drug for urticaria, so it should be used only in severe and refractory cases of CSU.

Other Alternatives

Montelukast
- No large-scale double-blind placebo-controlled study has been done with leukotriene receptor antagonists in CSU.
- The level of evidence for the efficacy of leukotriene receptor antagonists like montelukast in CSU is low and therefore, montelukast is not recommended routinely in the management of CSU.
- Leukotrienes receptor antagonists might have some role in patients whose urticaria is exacerbated by aspirin or other NSAIDs, although eliminating them, if possible, is a better approach.[1]

Dapsone
- Evidence is limited for the use of dapsone in CSU.
- The most recent trial demonstrated a response rate of 30–40% for dapsone, with a placebo response of 10%.[22]

H_2-antagonists
Though previously considered as a therapeutic option, H_2-antagonists are now perceived to have little evidence to maintain them as recommendable in the routine management of CSU but they may still have relevance as they are very affordable in some more restricted healthcare systems.[22]

Rare Treatment Options

Sulfasalazine, methotrexate, interferon, plasmapheresis, phototherapy, intravenous immunoglobulins (IVIG/IGIV) are other treatment options for CSU which have low-quality evidence but can be tried in selected case scenarios.[22]

Oral Corticosteroids

- A retrospective study of 750 patients states that 50% of patients with antihistamine-unresponsive CSU were successfully treated with a single course of prednisone starting with 25 mg/day and then tapered over 10 days.[23]
- In an Indian case series, 10 antihistamine-resistant CSU patients, treated for 2 months with methylprednisolone along with levocetirizine 5 mg daily caused a significant reduction in mean UAS7 scores.[24]
- However, keeping in mind the severe side effects associated with long-term use of corticosteroids, systemic steroids are recommended to be used sparingly only for a short duration of <7–10 days.[21]

Patient Education

Therapeutic patient education (TPE) allows patients to better understand their disease and cope with treatment. Studies have shown TPE improves knowledge and skills for CSU patients. Further research is needed to demonstrate the positive impact of TPE on CSU activity (**Table 2**).[25]

Treatment of Refractory Chronic Spontaneous Urticaria

For refractory CSU, drugs were tried beyond-label and off-label. Also, there are some novel therapeutics that can be promising in the management of CSU in the near future (**Fig. 3**).

TABLE 2: Standard therapeutic patient education questionnaire.	
What are hives?	Hives are raised, red, itchy rashes on the skin (also called wheals) Hives are often caused by an allergic reaction. The medical term for hives is urticaria
How do hives occur?	Episodes of hives may appear as a reaction to an allergen such as food or additives, medicine, or an insect bite or sting. Hives may also occur as a reaction to infection or emotional stress. However, often the cause of the hives cannot be determined
How long will the effects of hives last?	• The itching, swelling, and redness of hives can last hours to several weeks or months. In most cases, the hives eventually go away, but at least in a good proportion of patients hives can be recurrent or chronic • Chronic hives last a longer time. Most often it is not possible to determine their cause
How can I take care of myself?	• Take second-generation antihistamines or other medicines as prescribed by your healthcare provider to help relieve your symptoms • Avoid foods that seem to cause you to break out in hives • Visit your healthcare provider if you continue to have outbreaks of hives
What can I do to help prevent hives from recurring?	• If you know the cause of your hives, you should take steps to avoid the cause • You should take regular doses of antihistamine as suggested by your healthcare provider to prevent recurrences

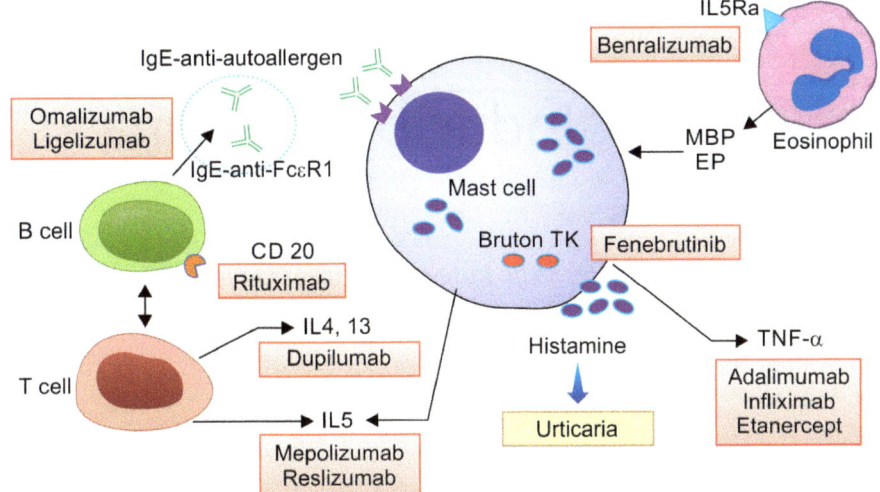

(CSU: chronic spontaneous urticaria; IL: interleukin; IgE: immunoglobulin E; TNF-α: tumor necrosis factor alpha)

FIG. 3: Targeted treatments for CSU.

Ligelizumab

- Ligelizumab is a humanized IgG1 monoclonal antibody that binds to the Cε3 domain of IgE with higher affinity than omalizumab.
- Ligelizumab provides greater and longer suppression of free IgE, basophil FcεRI, and basophil surface IgE in comparison to omalizumab. It has a faster onset of action and a superior dose-dependent efficacy over omalizumab.
- It also has a longer time to relapse after the last injection, i.e., 10 weeks versus 4 weeks with omalizumab.[4]

Dupilumab

Dupilumab, which is an effective treatment for atopic dermatitis, inhibits IL-4 and IL-13 effects through the blockade of their shared IL-4α receptor subunit. It was shown to benefit patients with refractory CSU unresponsive to omalizumab.[26]

Interleukin-5 Targeted Therapies

Anti-IL-5 receptor antibodies (benralizumab), and anti-IL-5 antibodies (mepolizumab and reslizumab) have been successfully used to treat patients with CSU.[27]

Bruton's Tyrosine Kinase Inhibitor

Treatment with Bruton's tyrosine kinase inhibitor (fenebrutinib and remibrutinib) inhibits IgE- and mast cell-mediated diseases including CSU.[27]

 ONLINE REFERENCES

To access the references of this chapter online, kindly refer to **emedicine360.com** also please follow the instructions mentioned on inside cover.

CHAPTER 5

Chronic Inducible Urticaria

Pelin Kuteyla CAN, Daria Fomina, Emek Kocatürk

INTRODUCTION

Chronic inducible urticaria (CIndU) is a subgroup of chronic urticaria characterized by recurrent itchy wheals and/or angioedema for longer than 6 weeks which occurs after exposure to certain eliciting trigger. CIndU is divided into two subtypes; physical [symptomatic dermographism (SD), cold and heat urticaria (HU), delayed pressure urticaria (DPU), solar urticaria (SU), and vibratory urticaria] and nonphysical urticarias [cholinergic urticaria (CholU), contact, and aquagenic urticaria (AqU)].[1-3] The estimated prevalence of CIndU is 0.5% in general population,[4] 5–25% among chronic urticaria and occurs most frequently in young adults.[5] Different from the CSU, CIndU has a long disease duration, and shorter lasting wheals.[4,6] The diagnosis of CIndU rely on history and should be confirmed by provocation testing (**Table 1**).[1]

TABLE 1: Features of inducible urticarias.

CIndU type	Clinical features	Trigger	Diagnostic test*[1,4]	Recommended laboratory test[2]
Symptomatic dermographism	Linear itchy wheals at the area of exposure (rubbing, scratching, scrubbing) (**Figs. 1A to C**)	Shear force (rubbing, scratching, scrubbing)	Moderate stroking of the skin on volar forearm or upper back with a blunt smooth object (e.g., closed ballpoint pen tip and wooden spatula), Fric test (longest pin) (**Figs. 1A**), or a dermographic tester (36 g/mm²) *Reading time*: 10 minutes after testing *Positive test*: Wheal and itch (**Figs. 1A and B**)	Differential blood count, ESR or CRP

Continued

Continued

CIndU type	Clinical characteristics	Trigger	Diagnostic test*[1,4]	Recommended laboratory test[2]
Cholinergic urticaria	Pinpoint wheals, with pronounced flare (**Fig. 1D**)	Active or passive body warming	*Exercise machines*: e.g., bicycle trainer or treadmill. Exercise for 30 minutes increase pulse rate by 3 beats/minute every minute, positive test = wheals. *If positive, wait > 24 hours and perform passive warming test* *A passive warming test*: 42°C bath, and monitor body temperature. Continue bath for 15 minutes after body temperature has increased by ≥1°C over baseline *Reading time*: During test as well as immediately and 10 minutes after end of test *Positive test*: Wheal	None
Cold urticaria	Occurrence of wheals upon exposure to cold or cooling stimuli (air, surfaces, objects or liquids) (**Fig. 1E**)	Cold air, objects, surfaces or liquids	*Ice cube testing*: Melting ice cube in thin plastic bag or TempTest (4–44°C) for 5 minutes on the volar forearm *Reading time*: 10 minutes after testing *Positive test*: Wheal (**Fig. 1F**)	Cryoglobulins,[4] infections screening
Delayed pressure urticaria	Cutaneous erythema and edema with often marked subcutaneous swelling after a pressure stimulus	Vertical pressure	Shoulder or upper back or thighs or volar forearm. Suspension of weights over shoulder (7 kg, shoulder strap width: 3 cm) for 15 minutes or weighted rods (1.5 cm diameter: 2.5 kg; or 6.5 cm diameter: 5 kg) for 15 minutes	None

Continued

Continued

CIndU type	Clinical characteristics	Trigger	Diagnostic test*[1,4]	Recommended laboratory test[2]
	Pressure-induced lesions typically occur 4–6 hours later, but may occur as early as 30 minutes and last up to 48 hours	Vertical pressure	Dermographic tester at 100 g/mm^2 for 70 seconds. Reading during 6 hours *Positive test*: Erythema and angioedema	
Heat urticaria	Appearance of wheals after contact with warm air, surfaces and liquids	Warm air, objects, surfaces or liquids	Heat source or TempTest (44–4°C) for 5 minutes on the volar forearm *Reading time*: 10 minutes after testing *Positive test*: Wheal	None
Solar urticaria	Sudden appearance of urticarial rash on areas of the skin that are exposed to light	Radiation spectrum from ultraviolet A to visible light (wavelength of 300–500 nm)	UVA 6 j/cm^2 and UVB 60 mj/cm^2 and visible light sources (projector) *Test site*: Buttocks *Reading time*: 10 minutes after testing *Positive test*: Wheal	None
Aquagenic urticaria	Small pruritic wheals surrounded by red halo (**Fig. 1G**)	Water, sweat, saliva, tears, high humidity	A compress or a towel soaked with 35–37°C water or physiological saline is placed on the patient's trunk. The compress or the towel can be taken off after 40 minutes or earlier, if the patient reports pruritus and first wheals are seen at the skin test site. The test is positive if urticarial lesions develop inside the contact area within 10 minutes after taking off the compress/towel	None

Continued

Continued

CIndU type	Clinical characteristics	Trigger	Diagnostic test*[1,4]	Recommended laboratory test[2]
Vibratory angioedema	Presence of itching and swelling at the site of skin expose to vibratory stimulation	Vibration, joking, clapping hands, vibratory machines	Vortex vibrator that is run 1000 rpm for 5 minutes on the volar forearm *Reading time*: 10 minutes after testing *Positive test*: Angioedema or wheal	None
Contact urticaria	Urticarial lesions after contact to an exogeneous agents	Contact with eliciting agent (i.e., latex, animal products, chemicals)	Using open controlled application testing, skin prick test, or closed patch tests for 20 minutes	None

*Antihistamines should be stopped at least 3 days before testing (allowing five plasma half-lives of drug elimination) and glucocorticosteroids 7 days before testing.

(CIndUs: chronic inducible urticarias; CRP: C-reactive protein; ESR: erythrocyte sedimentation rate)

SYMPTOMATIC DERMOGRAPHISM

Symptomatic dermographism (urticaria factitia and dermographic urticaria), the most common form of CIndU is characterized by itching and/or burning sensation and the development of linear wheals due to shear force on the skin, which can be due to scratching, rubbing or scrubbing (**Figs. 1A to C**).[1,4] The trunk and extremities are more commonly involved. SD may be provoked by scratching, after friction by a solid object, or tight clothes and bed sheets.[7] Whealing develops within seconds to minutes following the shear force acting on the skin and may persist for 1.5–2 hours, SD should be distinguished from simple dermographism, which is characterized as the transient dermographic wheal without itching.[4,5] SD occurs in approximately 1–5% of the population, frequently presenting in young adults.[1,5,8] The disease has a long course, and lasts for years.[1,4,5] Dermographism is generally idiopathic, it may be seen in people with diabetes, hyperthyroidism, hypothyroidism, menopause, pregnancy, or it can be medication-related such as penicillin, and SD may be triggered by infections such as bacterial, fungal infections, *Helicobacter pylori*, scabies, bites, and stress.[9,10] Diagnosis rely on history taking and provocation testing. Provocation testing can be performed by a blunt smooth object (e.g., closed ballpoint pen tip and wooden spatula), the Fric test (longest pin) (**Fig. 1A**), or a dermographic tester (36 g/mm^2)[1,11] (**Table 1**). Provocation testing confirms the diagnosis and assess trigger thresholds.[11]

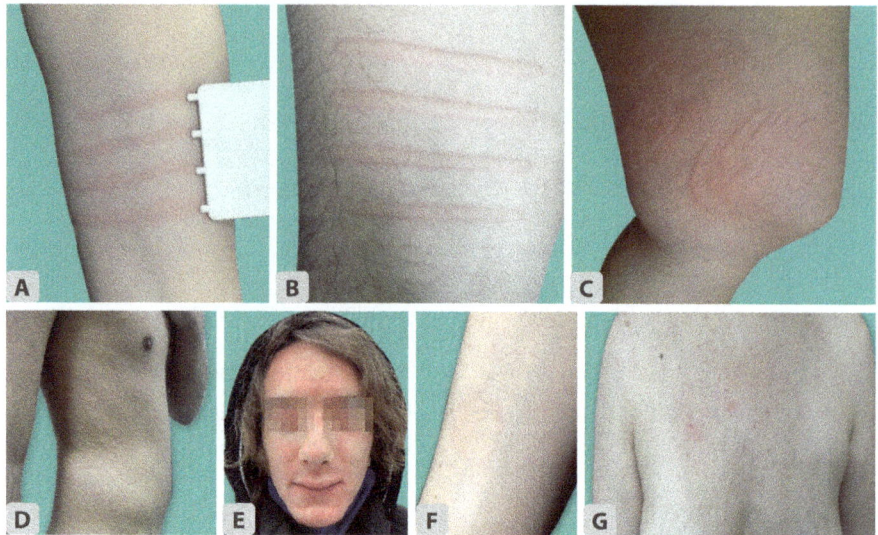

FIGS. 1A TO G: Features of different inducible urticarias. (A and B) symptomatic dermographism induced with Fric test 4.0 (positive result); (C) symptomatic dermographism; (D) cholinergic urticaria induced by exercise test; (E) cold urticaria; (F) cold urticaria induced by ice cube test (positive result); (G) aquagenic urticaria.

CHOLINERGIC URTICARIA

Cholinergic urticaria (CholU) is defined by itching, redness, and pinpoint sized papular whealing induced by a rise in body core temperature by active (e.g., exercise) or passive warming (e.g., hot bath). Other known triggers include sweating, hot baths or showers, eating of spicy foods or hot foods, and stress.[1,4,9,12] CholU initially presents as itchy pinpoint-sized (1-3 mm) urticarial eruptions surrounded by large flares usually localized to the trunk and proximal extremities (**Fig. 1D**),[12] but palms, soles, and axillae are spared.[13] Stinging or tingling sensations are present rather than itching in most of the cases.[13] Symptoms usually fade rapidly (15-60 minutes) on its own.[1,13] CholU may be accompanied by angioedema, respiratory symptoms and/or anaphylaxis.[13] CholU affects up to 4-11.2% of the population and mostly presents at the second or third decades.[1,12,13] Disease duration is 4-7.5 years and equal distribution for both sexes, or male predominance is reported.[1,14] Atopy, allergic rhinitis, and bronchial hyper-responsiveness can be seen more commonly in patients with CholU.[5,13] Exact etiology is not known yet, but histamine, cholinergic agents (e.g., acetylcholine), sweat allergy, serum factors, poral occlusion, and anhidrosis suggested to have a role in pathogenesis.[13] There are four subclasses reported due to assumed pathogenesis; (1) conventional sweat allergy-type, (2) follicular-type with a positive autologous serum skin test result, (3) CholU with palpebral angioedema, and (4) CholU with acquired anhidrosis and/or hypohidrosis.[5,13] Exercise induced anaphylaxis should be distinguished from CholU, which is an anaphylactic reaction induced by only physical activity, while patients with CholU manifest symptoms due to increase in body core temperature.[1,4] Provocation testing seems crucial (**Table 1**) to differentiate between these two entities.

COLD URTICARIA

Cold urticaria (ColdU) is characterized by the onset of symptoms upon contact with cold air, liquids or surfaces. The symptoms can range from erythema, itching, and wheals to angioedema (**Fig. 1E**) and in rare cases anaphylaxis can occur. These events significantly decrease patients' quality of life (QoL) and can be life-threatening.[15,16] ColdU can be either acquired or have autosomal dominant pattern of inheritance. The onset of acquired type often happens at a young age with the disease duration for 4–5 years, with subsequent remission or improvement in 50% of cases during 5 years.[17] The inherited type often has a childhood onset and accompanies patients throughout their life.[18] The prevalence is relatively equal among both sexes, the peak incidence occurs at a young age (18–27 years), ColdU can prevail in countries with a cold climate.[19] Overall estimated incidence of acquired ColdU in Central Europe is 0.05%.[17] The diagnosis is made according to the clinical symptoms, patient's medical history, and the provocation tests results (**Fig. 1F**) (**Table 1**). Further evaluation of the cryoglobulins levels and infections screening can be helpful. All patients should be thoroughly informed about the risks of life-threatening conditions and trained to avoid symptoms provoking factors—swimming in cold waters, eating cold foods/liquids, etc.

DELAYED PRESSURE URTICARIA

Delayed pressure urticaria (DPU) is characterized by the development of erythema and edema at the site of exposure to prolonged pressure on the skin. DPU differs from other forms of chronic idiopathic urticarias (CIUs) (with the exception of vibrational urticaria/angioedema) by the edema involvement of the deep layers of the dermis without wheals.[5,20]

The development of symptoms of DPU takes 4–6 hours on average remaining for 24 hours or more.[21,22] DPU is one of the least common types of CIU, occurring in <5% of cases of CIU.[23,24] The disease activity can vary depending on the time, on average it lasts from 6 to 9 years.[5,25]

Delayed pressure urticaria significantly deteriorates the patients' QoL mainly because it markedly limits activity associated with exposure to pressure (cycling, manual labor, prolonged standing or sitting), and affects the choice of clothing and shoes.[26] The rash/swelling can occur not only during work, associated with pressure, but it can also interrupt the natural routine of the patient (while walking, carrying weights, or during sexual intercourse). DPU is diagnosed according to medical history, and provocative pressure tests (**Table 1**).

Recommendations: To avoid symptom triggers such as specific activities, tight clothes and shoes, heavy bags, etc.

SOLAR URTICARIA

Solar urticaria (SU) is a chronic acquired disease associated with increased photosensitivity. It is characterized by the occurrence of wheals on the open areas of the body that have been exposed to sun. This disease is not life-threatening, but it can significantly limit daily activity and affect the QoL.[27-30]

Solar urticaria is a rare type of urticaria. It accounts for <0.5% of all cases of CIU and <7% of all photodermatoses. Mostly women are affected; the prevalence does not depend on ethnicity.[31,32] The symptoms often appear at a young age (under 35 years), the probability of spontaneous resolution of the disease was estimated as 15% after 5 years and 25% after 10 years of duration.[33] With prolonged sun exposure, angioedema of various localization may occur, in severe cases with systemic symptoms—weakness, headache, dizziness, nausea, etc. The diagnosis is established according to complaints and medical history (symptoms onset several minutes after solar exposure).

Recommendations: To avoid exposure to direct sunlight, to wear protective clothing, hats, sunglasses, accompanied by the sunscreen with a high protection index (SPF 50+).[4]

HEAT URTICARIA

Heat urticaria (HU) is one of the most rare types of CIndUs, characterized by itchy erythema and well-defined wheals that develop upon contact with warm objects/liquids,[2,34,35] two forms are defined—localized or generalized.[36]

Heat urticaria can be either acquired or hereditary with autosomal dominant pattern. Acquired HU is the most common one (82% of all cases), acute symptoms (wheals and/or angioedema) occur upon contact with a heat trigger and resolve in 1-3 hours.[37,38]

The onset of symptoms can occur with delay (in 0.5-2 hours) after a prolonged contact (12-14 hours) with heat triggers.[35,38] This form of HU is more typical for familial cases.[35] Patients with an immediate type of rash development can suffer from the angioedema predominantly localized on hands and face area.[39-41] In 53% of patients with HU the features of systemic reactions—weakness, dizziness, head and abdominal pain, nausea, vomiting, diarrhea, tachycardia, fever, as well as dyspnea, and syncope conditions can be registered. Patients should be informed about the potential life-threatening conditions, and trained to avoid trigger factors causing rash.

AQUAGENIC URTICARIA

Aquagenic urticaria (AqU) is a very rare form of CIndU.[1,42] AqU is characterized by 1-3 mm folliculocentric wheals with surrounding 1-3 cm erythematous flares (**Fig. 1G**) within 20-30 minutes following skin contact with any source of water at any temperature including sweat and tearsdiagnosis and management of CIndU.[1,42] Lesions fade within 30-60 minutes of cessation of water contact and skin lesions are associated with pruritus, burning, and prickling sensation. AqU mostly locates on the trunk and upper arms, while palms and soles are spared.[9,42] AqU develops during puberty, shows female predominance and has a chronic course.[9,43,44] It is mostly sporadic but can also be familial.[43,45] Systemic symptoms such as wheezing or shortness of breath are rarely reported.[1,42] CholU, aquagenic pruritus, ColdU, and HU should be differentiated from AqU by provocation testing (**Table 1**).[1,13,42,43]

VIBRATORY URTICARIA/ANGIOEDEMA

Vibratory urticaria/angioedema (VA), is a rare form of CIndU, which presents as erythematous wheals and/or angioedema on the skin which is exposed to vibration.[1,46,47] Common triggers are jogging, running, cycling, riding a motorcycle, horseback riding, massaging, working with machinery or cutting the grass.[46,47] Occupations that have the risk are; machinist, jackhammer operator, carpenter, and metal grinder operator[9,47] Patients feel itch or burning sensation at the skin sites where the vibration exposed to. Lesions occur within a few minutes following a vibratory stimulus and disappear within 24 hours. Delayed reactions (peak in 4-6 hours) and accompanying anaphylaxis were also reported. VA can be hereditary (HVA) and acquired (AVA).[9,46] HVA is less common than AVA, HVA has autosomal-dominant inheritance (mutation in the gene *ADGRE2*).[48] In HVA; positive family history, manifestation at birth, wheal formation, and systemic symptoms are more common than AVA, while history for atopy is rarer.[46]

CONTACT URTICARIA

Contact urticaria (CU) is characterized by the occurrence of a wheal and flare reaction of skin or mucosa within minutes (20-30 minutes) after contact to an offending agent and disappears within 24 hours.[47,49] CU is classified into immunologic (ICU), nonimmunologic (NICU), and indeterminate CU.[1,49] ICU is an allergic type I immunoglobulin E (IgE)-mediated hypersensitivity reaction that requires previous sensitization.[49,50] Lesion with central swelling, erythema, and warmth, surrounded by a peripheral pallor accompanied by pruritus is the clinical manifestation, angioedema may exist.[49] The reaction can spread and progress to generalized urticaria and even can lead systemic symptoms and anaphylactic shock, this step-wise progression is called as CU syndrome.[49-51] One of the most common triggers for ICU is latex but plant-derived proteins and, animal products, grains, enzymes, drugs, cosmetics, and chemicals can also induce ICU.[1,50,51] In contrast to ICU, NICU does not require previous sensitization and can occur at the first contact within 45 minutes up to an hour, lesions are limited to the area where the eliciting agents contact[1,49] and is mainly caused by low molecular weight agents (e.g., cinnamal, sorbic acid, benzoic acid aldehyde, and nicotinic acid esters), plants (e.g., stinging nettle), animals (e.g., jelly fish) can be the eliciting agents.[1,50] Greater reactions occur at face and back compared to the palms and soles. Prostaglandins and leukotrienes are mediators of NICU that is why it provide response to oral and topical nonsteroidal anti-inflammatory drugs.[49] Indeterminate CU can be both IgE-mediated and/or nonimmunologic, while exact pathophysiology is unknown. Ammonium persulfate (contained in hair bleaching products) is one example of agent that causes indeterminate CU.[49]

TREATMENT OF INDUCIBLE URTICARIA

Avoidance of the triggering factor or physical stimuli should be considered but it is not always possible, therefore pharmacological treatment is needed and treatment mainly aims to achieve complete symptom control. The recommended treatment approach in CIndU is the same as that for chronic spontaneous urticaria

(CSU).[2,52] Second-generation(sg) H_1-antihistamines (H_1-AHs) constitute the first line treatment in CIndU, when the standard doses of sg-AHs fails, increasing the dosage up to 4-folds should be recommended as second step. Half of the CIndU patients are H_1-AH resistant and, only third line treatment is omalizumab.[2,3,53] But omalizumab is still off-label for CIndU and there is a lack of clinical trials assessing efficacy of omalizumab in patients with CIndUs.[53,54] There are a few placebo controlled trials are available for SD, CholU, and ColdU, but real life studies and case series showed the efficacy of omalizumab in patients with CIndUs.[52,53,55-57] Nevertheless, there is need for more individualized treatment options which are more specific to the subtypes, since an important proportion of the patients are refractory to the available treatments. Critical threshold testing should be used to monitorize disease activity as well as the response to treatment.[1] Disease activity should be assessed before and during treatment to decide appropriate treatment step, however, threshold testing is not always possible.[2] Patient-reported outcome measures are important for measuring disease activity, disease control, and the impact of symptoms on patients' lives.[58] Dermatology life quality index (DLQI) may be used for QoL assessment and urticaria control test (UCT) can be used to assess the treatment response, if threshold testing cannot be performed.[2,11,58,59] There are few specific disease activity tools or QoL instruments available for CIndUs. Disease specific activity score (Chol-UAS) and QoL questionnaire (Chol-QoL) for CholU are available, and QoLs for ColdU (ColdU-QoL) and SD (SD-QoL) are under development.[4,6,60]

 ONLINE REFERENCES

To access the references of this chapter online, kindly refer to **emedicine360.com** also please follow the instructions mentioned on inside cover.

CHAPTER 6

Angioedema

Niall Conlon, I Boccon-Gibod, L Bouillet

INTRODUCTION

Angioedema (AE) refers to localized, episodic swelling of the skin, and mucous membranes. AE is the symptomatic end point of disparate pathological processes that result in increased vascular permeability and fluid accumulation in the subcutaneous and deep dermal layers of the skin or in the submucosa. AE is nonpitting to pressure, often asymmetric and can affect any part of the body.[1] This readily contrasts with the typically symmetrical involvement of pitting edema with its tendency to affect dependent peripheries.

For most patients, AE can lead to distressing, if temporary, disfigurement. Abdominal AE can be painful and involvement of the mouth and larynx can be terrifying and life-threatening. For nonspecialist clinicians a basic understanding of the main causes of AE will lead to a rational approach guided by the patient history that can inform timely investigation and effective management (**Fig. 1**).

MAST CELL ANGIOEDEMA

Mast cell angioedema (MC-AE) is often, but not always, accompanied by other features suggestive of mast cell activation. In its varied forms this type of AE is characterized by a response to histamine blockade. Above licensed doses of nonsedating antihistamines are often required, and sometimes other supportive therapies including glucocorticoids and epinephrine are needed.

Angioedema may be a life-threatening feature of anaphylaxis. Anaphylaxis, a rapidly evolving life-threatening allergic reaction, is due in part to histamine release from mast cells. This can result in AE accompanied by urticaria alongside cardiovascular and respiratory compromise.[2] Anaphylaxis is temporally associated with exposure to a culprit allergen. An allergy focussed clinical history is key in identifying suspect triggers and guiding selection of tests that may confirm allergic sensitization. Acute AE, again temporally related to an allergic trigger, may be a component of less severe allergic reactions that do not meet the definition of anaphylaxis. Anaphylaxis is a medical emergency requiring airway and circulatory support where required alongside rapid administration of intramuscular epinephrine, antihistamines, bronchodilators, and intravenous (IV) fluids may all be administered as part of supportive care. Identification and avoidance of the

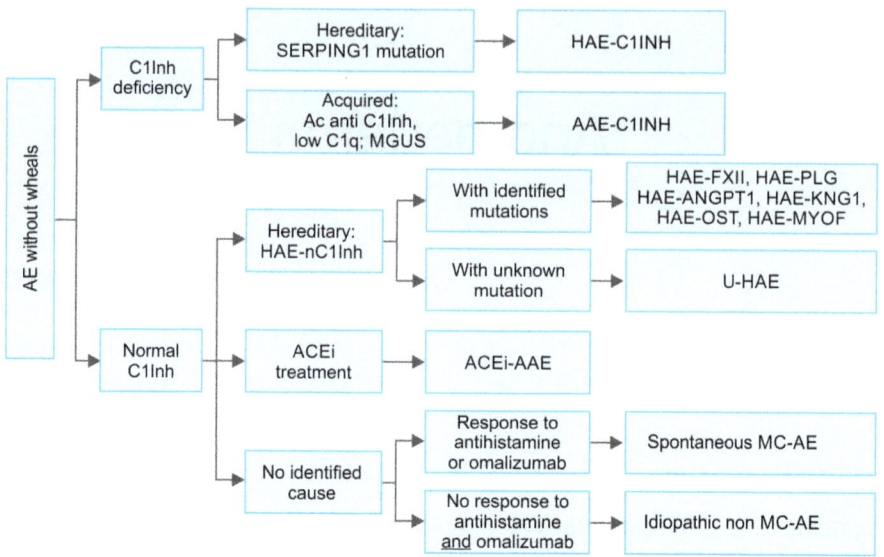

(AAE: acquired angioedema; AE: angioedema; ACE: angiotensin converting enzyme; C1Inh: C1 inhibitor; HAE: hereditary angioedema; MC: mast cell; MGUS: monoclonal gammapathy of unknown signification)

FIG. 1: Etiologies of angioedema without wheals.

allergic trigger is of paramount importance. A well-documented allergy clinical history taken immediately after the event can be invaluable in guiding subsequent investigation by allergists.

Mast cell angioedema is also frequently seem in the context of chronic spontaneous urticaria (CSU). CSU is defined as the presence of urticaria (hives) and/or AE (swellings) for 6 weeks or more. AE is present in 30–50% of cases. This condition is more common in females and affects all ages, although it presents more commonly in middle age. Patients typically report unpredictable symptoms without consistent relationships to foods, medications or other allergic triggers.[3]

Finally, MC-AE may be isolated and spontaneous. Spontaneous MC-AE is not accompanied by urticaria and lacks a plausible allergic explanation or drug trigger. The majority of such cases respond to antihistamines and are likely to represent a group that overlaps considerably with CSU, with identical management approaches. A minority of cases of isolated AE do not respond to histamine blockade and omalizumab.[4] These refractory patients may have bradykinin-mediated disease.

The management of AE in the context of chronic spontaneous urticaria angioedema (CSUA) or isolated spontaneous MC-AE is supported by evidence based guidelines.[3] These straightforward approaches based on the use of regular second generation antihistamines at normal and high (×4 licensed) doses are adequate to control many patients. Treatment resistant cases are managed with the anti-IgE monoclonal antibody omalizumab. In some countries access to omalizumab can be challenging. In this setting, agents such as cyclosporine may be considered. These older agents are now used less frequently. Novel emerging therapies may result in further reductions in the use of medications with challenging side effect profiles. A rational evidence based approach to the management of CSU and MC-AE has revolutionized the management of these conditions.

BRADYKININ-MEDIATED ANGIOEDEMA

Bradykinin-mediated angioedema (BK-AE) is a disparate but related family of disorders in which vascular permeability is driven primarily by BK release. Distinguishing BK-mediated from MC-AE can be challenging. A focussed clinical history and appropriate testing can often differentiate between the two groups of conditions. This is vital as some data suggests that mortality, while uncommon, is much higher in BK-AE and management strategies differ considerably between the two conditions.[5]

ANGIOTENSIN-CONVERTING ENZYME INHIBITOR INDUCED ANGIOEDEMA

Angiotensin-converting enzyme (ACE) inhibitor-angioedema is an uncommon, potentially fatal, complication of ACEi treatment.[6] AE due to ACE inhibitors is the second most common side effect of this therapy (after cough) with an estimated incidence between 0.1 and 0.7%. While ACE inhibitor-AE is a relatively unusual side effect of treatment, the widespread use of these agents mean that it is a common presentation to AE specialists. Although it most commonly occurs in the first 6 weeks of treatment, 20% of cases occur outside this initial phase. Indeed, AE can occur after many years of uneventful therapy when the index of suspicion of the prescriber is low.[7]

Angiotensin-converting enzyme inhibitor exert their therapeutic effects by blocking the conversion of angiotensin I to angiotensin II by ACE. ACE is also involved in the catabolism of BK. ACE inhibitor therapy can facilitate the accumulation of BK and the saturation of secondary degradation pathways.[8] Bradykinin exerts its pathological effect via BK2 receptors resulting in AE with a predilection for the face and upper airway that can be severe and life-threatening.

The acute management of ACE inhibitor-AE remains controversial. Despite initial promise, targeted treatments including icatibant and ecallantide have proven disappointing in appropriately powered clinical trials.[9,10] There is still some rationale and case report support for the use of C1 esterase inhibitor concentrate in severe cases but further study is required.[11,12] In practice, effective airway management, where appropriate, and supportive therapy facilitates resolution of most acute episodes.[2] The most important subsequent step is the identification of ACE inhibitor therapy as a significant cause or contributing factor to AE and discontinuing this treatment, irrespective of the duration of therapy.

It is vital to acknowledge that some patients – close to 50% in some studies, will have a recurrence of AE after the ACE inhibitor is discontinued.[4] In many such cases spontaneous MC-AE is the cause and is only diagnosed after a trial of regular treatment including antihistamines or in refractory cases anti-IgE therapy. Irrespective of this fact the discontinuation of ACE inhibitor therapy is vital as AE is an absolute contraindication to this treatment as there is a potential to exacerbate AE severity irrespective of the cause. The choice of angiotensin receptor blockers (ARBs) as a replacement for ACE inhibitor treatment has continued to be examined, however, most evidence suggests that ARBs do not increase AE risk.[13]

HEREDITARY ANGIOEDEMA DUE TO C1 INHIBITOR DEFICIENCY

Hereditary angioedema (HAE) is a rare genetic condition beloved by those composing questions for medical examinations. Affecting 1/50,000 individuals, AE in this setting is caused by accumulation of BK due to impaired regulation of the contact and kallikrein–kinin pathways. Urticaria is not present in these conditions and its presence essentially excludes the diagnosis and the requirement for assessment of C1 inhibitor. However, erythema marginatum, a rash that is typically nonpruritic may precede AE attacks in some individuals by several hours.

Hereditary angioedema is inherited in an autosomal dominant fashion and is due to mutations in the *SERPING1* gene.[14] Type 1 HAE is due to defective C1 inhibitor synthesis reflected by low serum levels and represents around 85% of cases. In type 2 HAE C1 inhibitor levels are normal but the enzyme is functionally defective with identical clinical consequences. A strong family history of AE is often readily elicited but de novo mutations can occur in 20% of cases. In addition, 15% of patients with the mutation are asymptomatic.

While a rare diagnosis and one of the less common causes of AE-it is straightforward and prudent to exclude C1 inhibitor deficiency in patients presenting with isolated AE without an obvious cause.[2] A low C4, caused by impaired C1 inhibitor regulation of the classical complement cascade, is often observed. However, it is not a universally sensitive screening tool and C4 levels may be normal between attacks. Measurement of both C1 inhibitor levels and function is recommended. Specimens for C1 inhibitor function can degrade rapidly and good communication with the referral laboratory is of paramount importance to prevent false results suggesting reduced activity. Abnormal test results should always be confirmed by repeat and interpreted in the light of the clinical history.

Hereditary Angioedema with Normal C1 Inhibitor

Hereditary angioedema with normal C1 inhibitor (HAE-n C1Inh) represents a significant diagnostic challenge. This very rare autosomal dominant condition is characterized by a strong family history of AE predominantly affecting females and often with evidence of marked estrogen sensitivity. Consensus criteria for diagnosis recommend the exclusion of significant C1 inhibitor abnormalities and excluding a response to high dose antihistamines (and omalizumab). The identification in 2006 of mutations in *F12* coding for factor XII provided an explanation for some of these cases. Since then disease causing variants have been identified in other genes (*ANGPT1, KNG1, PLG, XPNPEP1, 3-OST-6,* and *MYOF-217S*) coding for proteases and protease inhibitors of the kallikrein–kinin and fibrinolytic pathways.[15] The lack of robust biomarkers and challenges accessing genetic tests might suggest underdiagnosis of these conditions internationally.

Acquired C1 Inhibitor Deficiency

The acquisition of C1 inhibitor deficiency later in life is rare but well described. Patients usually present after the age of 40 years. Levels of C4 and C1 inhibitor protein or function are reduced to <50%.[16] Reduced levels of C1q are a useful discriminatory biomarker of acquired C1 inhibitor deficiency. The pathomechanism of acquired C1 inhibitor deficiency may be related to excess consumption due to complement activation or due to the production of a functional autoantibody directed against C1 inhibitor. Cases may be linked to autoimmune diseases such as systemic lupus erythematosus or lymphoproliferative disorders including monoclonal gammopathy of undetermined significance.[16] Importantly, acquired C1 inhibitor deficiency may precede the diagnosis of lymphoproliferative disease by several years so close follow up is warranted. Where an underlying disorder is identified treatment of this may alleviate AE symptoms.

Idiopathic Nonmast Cell Angioedema

This is a relatively commonly encountered outcome following careful exclusion of other causes of AE and treatment with high dose antihistamines.[4] Nonmast cell AE remains poorly explored. Evidence from case series supports the trial of anti-IgE therapy in such cases. Failure suggests, but does not confirm, a BK-mediated disorder. The optimal management of such cases requires further clarification but may include tranexamic acid or BK receptor blockers.

Treatments for Bradykinin-mediated Angioedema

Aside from ACE inhibitor-AE, BK-AE including the various forms of HAE and AAE should be managed in expert centers. Details of the guideline driven management for these conditions is beyond the scope of this chapter. Replacement of C1 inhibitor with infusions of C1 inhibitor concentrate or blockade of BK by the subcutaneous B2 receptor antagonist icatibant is effective in the management of acute BK-AE attacks.[17,18] Home possession facilitating "on-demand" treatment using such agents has helped patients reduce the requirement for emergency department attendance and improved quality of life. Progress has been made too with prophylactic agents to reduce the frequency of attacks. Traditionally used medications include tranexamic acid, an antifibrinolytic with little supportive evidence, and attenuated androgens that can have unacceptable side effects are still used. However, high quality evidence demonstrating the impact of a number of agents has been developed over recent years. Regular IV or subcutaneous infusions of C1 inhibitor concentrate are effective. The subcutaneous recombinant monoclonal kallikrein inhibitor lanadelumab is now widely licensed for long-term prophylaxis.[19] Recently, the Food and Drug Administration (FDA) approved the first oral kallikrein inhibitor, berotralstat for use in preventing HAE attacks.[20] Accessing these new and effective treatments will be a significant challenge for specialists in these area.

CONCLUSION

An understanding of the principles of MC and BK-mediated AE is useful for physicians across a range of specialties. Attention to a focused clinical history can direct appropriate testing and early effective management.

ONLINE REFERENCES

To access the references of this chapter online, kindly refer to **emedicine360.com** also please follow the instructions mentioned on inside cover.

CHAPTER 7

Urticaria and Comorbidities

*Maia Gotua, Rosana Câmara Agondi,
Ivan Cherrez Ojeda*

INTRODUCTION

Urticaria is a mast cell (MC) driven skin disease and the degranulation of this cell is triggered by the activation of several receptors on its surface. All MC express high-affinity immunoglobulin E (IgE) receptors (FcεRI) and, increasingly, the IgE-FcεRI complex appears to be involved in the autoimmune etiology of chronic spontaneous urticaria (CSU), through the presence of IgG anti-FcεRI/anti-IgE or IgE against autoallergens.[1,2]

Besides FcεRI-IgE complex, MC expresses numerous G protein-couple receptors (GPCRs), which are the largest group of membrane receptor proteins. Several drugs, antimicrobial host defense peptides, neuropeptides, major basic protein, eosinophil peroxidase, among other substances activate this type of receptor.[3,4] *MRGPRX2* receptor on MCs, basophils, and eosinophils associated with IgE-independent degranulation, has been reported to be highly expressed on cutaneous MCs in patients with severe CSU.[5]

Mast cells are multifunctional cells presented throughout the body and play important role in the maintenance of many physiological functions as well as in the pathophysiology of different diseases (allergy, asthma, anaphylaxis, gastrointestinal disorders, many types of malignancies, and cardiovascular diseases).[5,6] MCs association with autoimmune diseases (AIDs) includes multiple sclerosis, rheumatoid arthritis, insulin-dependent diabetes mellitus, bullous pemphigoid, chronic idiopathic urticaria (CIU), experimental vasculitis, autoimmune thyroid disease, etc.[7,8]

Comorbidities mean the presence of one or more additional diseases or disorders occurring concomitantly with a primary disease or disorder. Comorbidities can add layers of complexity and often lead to a worse prognosis for the underlying disease. Managing comorbidities is challenging, one condition can contribute or be linked to another and treatments can act synergistically, or conflict with each other and modify the response to the drugs used to control diseases.[9]

There are certain comorbidities, frequently associated with urticaria: Autoimmunity, infections, atopic/allergic diseases, emotional stress/psychiatric disorders, and metabolic syndrome (MetS) with dietary factors that can aggravate chronic urticaria (CU), etc.[1,2,10-19] Some patients have even not one, but several multiple comorbidities. These patients are older, had longer urticaria duration and are more refractory to antihistamines, which may indicate worse prognosis. The progressive increase in the number of comorbidities, in the same patient, favors the hypothesis of CU to behave as a low-grade systemic inflammatory disease.[20]

URTICARIA AND AUTOIMMUNITY

Indirect evidence for CU being an autoimmune disease comes from an observed association with other AIDs, a strong association between serum functionality and human leukocyte antigen (HLA)-DR4 haplotype and the good response of CU patients to immunotherapies.[21] Many studies in different populations indicate that CSU is strongly linked to various AIDs, primarily Hashimoto's thyroiditis (HT), vitiligo, pernicious anemia, Graves' disease, type 1 diabetes mellitus, rheumatoid arthritis, psoriasis, celiac disease, systemic lupus erythematosus, Sjögren syndrome, inflammatory bowel disease, Henoch–Schönlein purpura, and Kawasaki disease.[2,22-27] Patients with CSU are at risk of AIDs, especially adult female patients with a positive family history and a genetic predisposition for autoimmune disorders, who should be screened for signs and symptoms of common AIDs, especially HT and vitiligo.[2,22] CSU often precedes the onset of other AIDs.[23,26,28-30]

Over the past years, two groups of MC-degranulating signals have been identified and characterized: IgE autoantibodies to autoallergens and autoantibodies that target activating MC receptors. According to this two endotypes of CSU have been recently proposed: *Autoallergic* and *autoimmune*, the first is defined as type I autoimmune CSU mediated by IgE autoantibodies *(TIaiCSU)* and the second—*aiCSU*, defined as type IIb autoimmune CSU *(TIIbaiCSU)* in which IgG autoantibodies, and in addition to IgG, IgM, and IgA are responsible for direct activation of MC through binding to high-affinity IgE receptors.[1,2,31,32] Thyroperoxidase (TPO) has been demonstrated to be a common and relevant autoallergen in *TIaiCSU*, beyond TPO there are IgE autoantibodies directed to another autoantigens: Thyroglobulin, tissue factor, and interleukin-24 (IL-24).[1,29]

According to Maurer M et al. 2020 there is a strong evidence that total IgE is currently one of the best generally available surrogate marker for the routine diagnostic workup of CSU patients and discrimination of TIaiCSU and TIIbaiCSU.[1,31] Altrichter S et al. showed that high total IgE levels may indicate to TIaiCSU, high disease activity, longer disease duration, a high chance to respond to omalizumab therapy, quick relapse after stopping omalizumab, and a lower chance of responding to cyclosporine.[31] The assessment of pre- and posttreatment IgE levels and their ratio may help to diagnose and improve the management of TIaiCSU patients who require omalizumab treatment.[33] TIIbaiCSU accounts 8% of CSU patients,[28] they are characterized with markedly lower total IgE levels, expressed markers for AIDs, antinuclear antibodies (ANAs) and/or IgG antithyroid antibodies[2] with decreased probability to respond to omalizumab and a better chance to benefit from cyclosporine treatment.[31] These patients have higher rates of eosinopenia and basopenia,[1] highly expressed *MRGPRX2* receptor on cutaneous MC, especially in patients with severe CSU.[5] Schoepke N et al.[28] recommended to use the ratio of IgG anti-TPO to total IgE, as marker for TIIbaiCSU. The current gold standard for the diagnosis of TIIbaiCSU are: Positive autologous serum skin test (ASST); basophil histamine release assay (BHRA), and immunoassay for specific IgG autoantibodies against FcεRIα/IgE.[21]

A systematic analysis of autoimmune comorbidity by Kolkhir P et al. 2017, in CSU revealed, that the rates of comorbidity in most studies were ≥1% for insulin-dependent diabetes mellitus, rheumatoid arthritis, psoriasis, and celiac disease, ≥2% for Graves' disease, ≥3% for vitiligo, and ≥5% for pernicious anemia and HT.[22] More than 15% of CSU patients had a positive family history for AIDs.[2,26] The prevalence of hives in AID patients was noted in >1% of most studies.[22] Hypothyroidism and HT are more common than hyperthyroidism and Graves' disease in patients with CSU and correspondingly, elevated levels of IgG against TPO are often observed in those patients.[23,26]

Recently, Kolkhir P et al. 2021, showed that 28% of CSU patients had at least 1 AID, mostly HT (≥21%) and vitiligo (2%).[2] Around 2% of CSU patients had ≥2 AIDs predominantly combination of above the mentioned diseases.

URTICARIA AND INFECTIOUS DISEASES

Helicobacter pylori (HP) has been considered to be associated with the occurrence and persistence of CSU.[34,35] The meta-analysis of Kim HJ et al. 2019 confirmed the evident benefit of HP eradication in suppressing CSU symptoms, however, there was no significant difference in the remission of CSU whether antibiotic therapy was successful in eradication of HP or not.[35] Further studies are recommended to explore the mechanisms of comorbidities of HP with CSU.

Some parasites: Toxocara, fasciola, ancylostoma, strongyloides, filaria, echinococcus, trichinella, Schistosoma mansoni, Blastocystis hominis, etc., all have been associated with acute urticaria.[36] *Anisakis simplex* can also cause urticaria after eating of contaminated sushi fish with the parasites.[37]

Epidemiological studies and case reports suggest that some bacterial, fungal, and viral infections might be associated with the CSU, they are: *Streptococcus, Staphylococcus, Mycoplasma pneumoniae, Salmonella, Brucella, Borrelia, Chlamydia pneumonia, Yersinia enterocolitica,* herpesviridae, parvoviridae, caliciviridae, picornaviridae, flaviviridae, hepadnaviridae, etc.[38,39]

Chronic viral infections, including hepatitis B and C, have been reported to be associated with CSU, correspondingly patients with CSU have markers of hepatitis B (<5%) and C (2%). Urticarial rash occurs in ≤3% of patients with hepatitis C.[40]

More research is needed to assess the role of infections in pathogenesis of CSU. The routine screening of parasitic, bacterial or viral infections in CU is not recommended, however, testing a patient with urticaria for certain infections is a physician's choice based on the specific characteristics of the patient, and such are clinical symptoms and laboratory results, dietary and cultural habits, country of origin and residency, traveling history.[41]

The coronavirus disease 2019 (COVID-19) pandemic dramatically disrupts health care around the globe. Cutaneous manifestations are prevalent and on occasions can be the first presenting symptom for COVID-19 infection, for example severe urticarial rash as the initial symptom of COVID-19.[42]

The impact of the pandemic on CU and its management was analyzed by Kocaturk et al. 2021, in urticaria centers of reference and excellence (UCARE) COVID-CU study.[42] It was concluded that the COVID-19 pandemic severely impairs CU patient care resulting in <50% reduction of numbers of weekly treated patients, due to restricted patients' referrals in clinics and decreased clinic hours. This study revealed that CU does not affect the course of COVID-19, but COVID-19 results in CU exacerbation in one of three patients, with higher rates in patients with severe COVID-19.[43]

URTICARIA AND ATOPIC/ALLERGIC DISEASES

Type I immediate IgE-mediated allergic reactions often involve acute urticaria after exposure to the culprit allergen. These causes include foods and food additives, medications (beta-lactams/penicillins, cephalosporins, and other drugs), insect stings and bites, latex, and blood products. Allergic reactions may be presented by the skin manifestations, or may be a part of a systemic allergic reaction (e.g., anaphylaxis). Generalized urticaria/angioedema following exposure to a causative allergen should be interpreted as a systemic reaction with a potential risk of anaphylaxis after subsequent exposure.[44]

Certain drugs (narcotics, muscle relaxants, vancomycin, and radiocontrast media), foods (tomatoes, strawberries, etc.), and plants (stinging nettle—*urtica dioica*) can cause urticaria due to MC degranulation through a nonIgE-mediated mechanism.[45]

Nonsteroidal anti-inflammatory drugs (NSAIDs) can trigger urticaria and/or angioedema by two distinct mechanisms: Due to underlying abnormalities in arachidonic acid metabolism (aspirin exacerbated cutaneous and/or respiratory disease) and allergic reactions to NSAIDs, that may be both very severe.[46]

IgE-mediated type I allergic reactions are extremely rare causes of CSU, on another hand, pseudoallergic (nonallergic hypersensitivity reactions) to NSAIDs or food may be more relevant for CSU.[1,46]

The highest levels of IgE were found in atopic patients with CSU,[30] CSU with concomitant gastroesophageal reflux disorder,[13] and CSU patients with high IL-33 serum levels.[47] Patients with a severe CSU had higher IL-17 and IL-33 levels, in comparison with mild disease, while pruritus severity has been associated with higher levels of IL-31.[47] Elevated levels of multifunctional key cytokines of inflammation and immunity-IL-17, IL-31, and IL-33 among CSU patients indicate a functional role of these cytokines in the pathogenesis of CSU.[47] On another hand, IL-33/IL-31 axis represents a potential pathway of inflammation in allergic and AIDs and explains their comorbidities with CSU.[48]

According to systematic analysis of comorbidities of CSU in children <12 years old the prevalence of atopy was 28.1% (15.4%—asthma, 13.08%—allergic rhinitis, and 9.4%—atopic dermatitis), autoimmunity was detected with the positive ASST in 36.8%, ANA-10.4%, and anti-TPO/antithyroglobulin (anti-TG) antibodies in 6.4%, while seroprevalence for HP in 21.1%, low vitamin D level in 69.1%, and psychiatric disorders in 70.4%.[49]

URTICARIA AND METABOLIC SYNDROME

Urticaria and MetS are associated with cardiovascular disease including the increased risk for coronary heart disease and other forms of cardiovascular atherosclerotic diseases. MetS includes glucose intolerance, dyslipidemia, hypertension, and central obesity. This syndrome is a complex disorder with high socioeconomic cost, moreover, it is considered as a worldwide epidemic.[14] Ye YM et al.[18] observed that 30% of patients with CU also had MetS, and this comorbidity was associated with a more severe and uncontrolled CU.

In a literature review, authors showed that MetS is becoming increasingly valued in patients with autoimmune skin diseases, including CU. They concluded that immunologic, metabolic, genetic, and environmental factors play an important role in the pathophysiology of several cutaneous diseases and that chronic inflammation may explain the link between autoimmune disease and MetS.[16]

Shalom et al.[19] investigated the association between CU and MetS and its components, obesity, hypertension, hyperlipidemia, and diabetes, in a large community-based healthcare database. This was a cross-sectional study that included 11,261 patients with CU and matched 67,216 controls. In this study, patients were predominantly young women. The authors found that CU was significantly associated with MetS and its components: Diabetes, obesity, hyperlipidemia, and hypertension. This observation was in line with the growing concept of CU as a chronic low-grade inflammatory condition and has clinical applications in the public health point of view. Early detection and treatment of MetS or its components in patients with CU may prevent its complications. Authors suggested that clinicians should take into account that patients with CU may need screening for MetS in the appropriate clinical settings.[19]

URTICARIA, EMOTIONAL STRESS, AND PSYCHIATRIC DISEASES

In CSU patients, relapses of symptoms of wheals, angioedema or both for several times a week, or even daily have a troublesome impact on their quality of life (QoL) and psychological state. CU belongs to a group of psychodermatological disorders accompanied by itch that may be a source of distress (anxiety, depression, and somatoform disorders) and could worsen patients' QoL.[50-54] Emotional stress is an important trigger and risk factor for psychiatric disorders, which is represented in >30% of patients with CSU. Screening for psychological health problems among CSU patients should be a necessity.[50]

In the systematic review of the literature and meta-analysis Konstantinou GN et al. 2019, showed that almost one out of three CU patients had at least one underlying psychiatric disorder.[50] The most prevalent psychiatric disorders were sleep-wake disorders, followed by anxiety, mood, trauma and stress-related disorders, somatic symptoms and related disorders, obsessive-compulsive and related disorders, and substance-related and addictive disorders, varying from 4 to 36.7% independent of whether studies had a control group.[50] In the same study no definite association was found between pre-existence of psychiatric disorders and the CU onset, no correlation was found between CU severity and duration, and psychological functioning.[50]

Tat TS, 2019. detected higher levels of depression and anxiety in patients with CSU.[51] The depression and anxiety assessed by the hospital anxiety and depression scale was evident in almost half of the 50 CSU patients with a significant positive correlation of both with the urticaria activity score.[51] Patients with CSU often have sleep disorders (SDs) because of pruritus. However, SDs might also contribute to the development of CSU.[52]

Ograczyk-Piotrowska A et al. 2018, investigated impact of the stress and itch on QoL in CU females.[53] CU patients demonstrated a significantly higher stress level in comparison to the control group. Regarding the total pruritus score, all urticaria quality of life questionnaire (CU-Q2oL) dimensions were affected, except for subscale swelling/mental status.[53]

The elevated psychological stress level that has been closely related to CSU/CIU could be attributed to the imbalance or irregularity of the neuroimmunecutaneous complex, with numerous neuropeptides, neurokinins, inflammatory mediators and cells, hypothalamic-pituitary-adrenal axis hormones, and the skin, but it is still unclear and must be further investigated whether any psychological stress or psychiatric disorder results in, or triggers onset of CSU/CIU on the top of pre-existing neuroimmune dysregulation.[50]

In conclusion, further multidisciplinary studies are needed to clarify urticaria and comorbidity issues, explore mechanisms and biomarkers of these associations, assess whether other (e.g., malignancies, gastrointestinal, etc.), diseases coexist with CU for improving interventions, that may help in CU control.

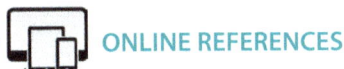 ONLINE REFERENCES

To access the references of this chapter online, kindly refer to **emedicine360.com** also please follow the instructions mentioned on inside cover.

CHAPTER 8

Role of Infections in Urticaria

Michael Rudenko

INTRODUCTION

The scientific evidence related to mast cells that was accumulated over the past 100 years, includes protective innate and adaptive immune responses to various pathogens and some infections.[1]

Clinical research in urticaria and angioedema is rapidly progressing.[2] A role of infection is being debated among leading the European Academy of Allergology and Clinical Immunology/Global Allergy and Asthma European Network/European Dermatology Forum/World Allergy Organization (EAACI/GA²LEN/EDF/WAO) scientists during the revision of guidelines, that are produced every 4 years by a global panel of experts.[3]

The role of viral and bacterial infections including coronavirus disease 2019 (COVID-19), herpes, viral hepatitis, and *Helicobacter Pylori*, in acute, acute-recurrent and chronic urticaria, and angioedema has been demonstrated in a number of original articles and case reports (**Fig. 1**). The disease activity can markedly change over time and is different between individual patients.[4]

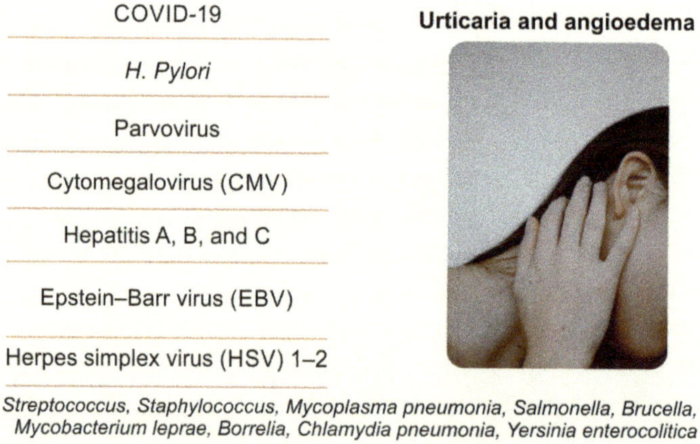

COVID-19	**Urticaria and angioedema**
H. Pylori	
Parvovirus	
Cytomegalovirus (CMV)	
Hepatitis A, B, and C	
Epstein–Barr virus (EBV)	
Herpes simplex virus (HSV) 1–2	

Streptococcus, Staphylococcus, Mycoplasma pneumonia, Salmonella, Brucella, Mycobacterium leprae, Borrelia, Chlamydia pneumonia, Yersinia enterocolitica

(COVID-19: coronavirus disease 2019; *H. pylori*: *Helicobacter pylori*)

FIG. 1: Infections that are described in literature in conjunction with urticaria and angioedema.

The EAACI/GA²LEN/EDF/WAO guidelines for the definition, classification, diagnosis, and management of urticaria indicate that various infections in urticaria can be either an underlying cause, an aggravating factor or not directly related condition. Many international organizations endorsed the document, including AAAAI, AAD, AAIITO, ACAAI, AEDV, APAAACI, ASBAI, ASCIA, BAD, BSACI, CDA, CMICA, CSACI, DDG, DDS, DGAKI, DSA, DST, EAACI, EIAS, EDF, EMBRN, ESCD, GA²LEN, IAACI, IADVL, JDA, NVvA, MSAI, ÖGDV, PSA, RAACI, SBD, SFD, SGAI, SGDV, SIAAIC, SIDeMaST, SPDV, TSD, UNBB, UNEV, and WAO.[3]

It was shown that eradication of a concomitant infection in some cases can lead to resolution of chronic urticaria and angioedema, but at present it is difficult to establish what are the mechanisms of this relationship in various infections?[5]

In routine clinical practice, it was noted that a history of bacterial infections, as well as viral, fungal or parasitic infections can be preceding an onset of chronic spontaneous urticaria.[6] The current guidelines recommend in the diagnostic process to focus on patient history for discovering potentially relevant infections, as well as laboratory tests including differential blood count analyses, determination of blood sedimentation rate, and C-reactive protein.[2]

Among patients with urticaria the rate of infections in a number of clinical trials was reported in the range of 37-58%.[7] It is believed that autoimmune nature of chronic spontaneous urticaria can be a leading factor in about 50% of persistent manifestations.[8]

Chronic spontaneous urticaria patients were shown to have elevated levels of specific immunoglobulin E (IgE) against a mix of *Staphylococcus aureus* enterotoxins in 51% of patients compared to 33% in healthy controls, when total serum IgE levels and disease activity in chronic spontaneous urticaria were correlated with *Staphylococcus* enterotoxin B-IgE levels.[9]

The current understanding of the underlying mechanisms of urticaria relates to increased permeability of blood vessels and irritation of nerve endings, leading to swelling and pruritus, following the activation of mast cells and basophils with release of proinflammatory mediators.[10]

At present we have to rely on data of case reports that showed association between acute urticaria and streptococcal infection,[11] hepatitis A[12] and B viruses,[13] parvovirus B19, cytomegalovirus (CMV),[14] coxsackie A9 virus,[15] enterovirus, influenza A[16] and parainfluenza viruses, and retrospective observational studies without appropriate controls that report evidence for a larger range of infectious agents triggering acute or recurrent acute urticaria and angioedema.[17]

Upper respiratory or digestive symptoms are common in urticaria associated with infections.[18] There were reports of *Mycoplasma pneumoniae* infection in 32% out of 65 children with acute urticaria.[19] There were observations of urticaria symptoms after influenza vaccination and more recently COVID-19 vaccinations.[16] Viral infection can be a potential trigger and sometimes the main etiologic agent in causing acute or chronic urticaria.[20]

The rates of hepatitis B and C infection do not appear to be increased in patients with chronic spontaneous urticaria and are only affecting <5% and 2% suggesting that viral hepatitis and chronic spontaneous urticaria are not usually linked,[21] although is being hypothesized that hepatitis B virus (HBV) and/or hepatitis C virus (HCV) infection may enhance IgE-induced mediator release from mast cells and basophils.[22] Human basophils and skin mast cells can be activated during viral hepatitis by protein Fv, leading to release histamine and other mediators.[23] The activation of mast cells can be induced by Fv protein that acts as an endogenous superantigen by interacting with the VH3 domain of IgE.[24]

It was shown that acute urticaria can be associated with infections caused by viruses of herpes group, and reactivation of herpes infection was associated with cutaneous urticarial-like syndromes, but there are not many data on reactivation of latent herpesvirus infections in association with chronic urticaria.[25]

There is a hypothesis that reactivation of a latent herpesviruses may play a role in chronic viral urticaria–that is suggested to have and underlying inflammatory process with autoimmune features.[25]

There as serological evidence in some patients with urticaria, showing increased immune response to human herpesvirus 4 (HHV-4) (Epstein–Barr virus, or EBV). These observations, combined with case reports of benefits of antiviral therapy leading to improvement of urticaria, suggest that viral infections might work as cofactors in chronic spontaneous urticaria. An observation that HHV-6 can potentially interact with HHV-4 in cutaneous layers, makes these viruses an interesting target for further research projects.[25]

COVID-19 outbreak was associated with self-reported urticaria among community-acquired cases in 1.4% of adult patients in Wuhan, China.[26]

From a series of 88 patients with an overall median age of 57.0 years 20% developed cutaneous manifestations including erythematous rash, widespread urticaria, and chickenpox like vesicles.[27]

In a later publication the rate of cutaneous manifestations of COVID-19 infection was in the form of a papulovesicular rash in 34.7%, (25/72) and urticaria in 9.7%, (7/72).[28]

The publication, produced but Urticaria Centers of Reference and Excellence (UCARE) from around the Globe, concludes that chronic urticaria does not appear to affect the course of COVID-19, but COVID-19 results in urticaria exacerbation in one of three patients. COVID-19 in more than a third of patients (36%), resulted in urticaria exacerbation, and exacerbations were more common in patients hospitalized due to COVID-19 infection.[29]

Viral infections in acute or chronic urticaria might serve as potential triggers and sometimes as the main etiologic factor. Manifestations of urticaria resolve or improve after the resolution or achievement of control of the concomitant viral infections.[30]

There are reports of association of various infections with urticaria and angioedema, they include *Helicobacter Pylori*,[31] *Streptococcus*,[13] *Staphylococcus*,[9] *Mycoplasma pneumonia*,[19] *Salmonella, Brucella, Mycobacterium leprae, Borrelia, Chlamydia pneumoniae,* and *Yersinia*.[11]

Urticaria, might be associated with release of bacterial toxins, presence of microorganisms in the areas of the skin with superficial damage, and accumulation of circulating immune complexes resulting in activation of components of complement.[5]

Helicobacter Pylori infection might be a risk factor for development of chronic urticaria. Further research of correlation between *H. Pylori* and urticaria may help clinicians to find more effective methods to treat people with chronic urticaria.[20] Detection of anti–*H. Pylori* IgG antibodies demonstrated that seropositivity was higher in the urticaria patients, comparing to a control group. Stool test for *H. Pylori* antigen is recommended in the diagnostic workup.[32] *H. Pylori* is a spiral-shaped microaerophilic gram-negative bacterium that colonizes the gastric mucosa and induces strong inflammatory response with various bacterial and host-dependent cytotoxic substances.[33]

According to meta-analysis there was a significant correlation of effective *H. Pylori* eradication therapy and favorable outcome in chronic spontaneous urticaria, leading to suggestion that *H. Pylori* might be associated with the occurrence and persistence of urticaria. Interestingly, according to the authors the resolution of chronic spontaneous urticaria was not associated with effectiveness of eradication treatment of *H. Pylori* infection, showing that following antibiotic therapy the patients showed significantly higher rate of remission of urticaria with or without successful *H. Pylori* eradication.[31]

Recurrent sinusitis or tonsillitis—bacterial infections of the nasopharynx can be diagnosed by using a range of tools: Antistreptolysin test for streptococcal or test for staphylococcal infection, imaging, with co-operation with different specialists including dentists and ENT consultants.[34]

Further research is required to explain the mechanisms of interaction between infections and urticaria and angioedema. The current working hypothesis is that the underlying immune response to an infection, rather than infection itself is the causative factor for persistence of urticaria alongside with the autoimmune factors. Antibodies and co-factors acting together reduce the threshold of reactivity leading to activation of mast cells.

We need to give answers to many unanswered questions, develop routine diagnostic tests that will help to detect underlying causes for urticaria and angioedema, arrange the global dissemination and consistent use of tools to assess disease activity, impact, and control, and develop more effective and well-tolerated long-term treatments for all forms of urticaria and angioedema.

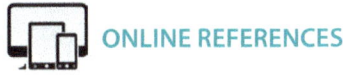 ONLINE REFERENCES

To access the references of this chapter online, kindly refer to **emedicine360.com** also please follow the instructions mentioned on inside cover.

CHAPTER 9

Differential Diagnosis

*Mojca Bizjak, Krzysztof Rutkowski,
Margarida Gonçalo*

INTRODUCTION

Urticaria is a disease that presents with mast cell-mediated wheals, angioedema, or both. It can be acute or chronic urticaria (CU); spontaneous or inducible. Chronic spontaneous urticaria (CSU) is the most common underlying disease in patients with recurrent wheals for >6 weeks.[1] It is usually a straightforward diagnosis, but there are several diseases that may mimic it. *Wheals* are transient, skin colored or erythematous, superficial, usually itchy, relatively soft, smooth papules or plaques (**Figs. 1** to **5**).

They occur rapidly due to dermal edema and completely resolve within 30 minutes to 24 hours, but new wheals may develop at other sites. This can be confirmed by marking a few skin lesions with a pen and then reviewing them in the following 24 hours (**Fig. 2**). CSU wheals may be round, oval, annular (ring-shaped) or polycyclic (connected rings; **Fig. 3**) and measure from a few millimeters to large,

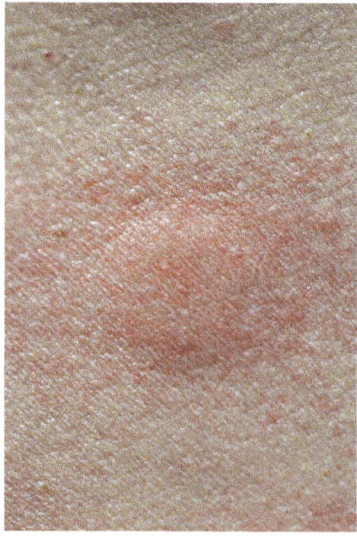

FIG. 1: Spontaneous wheal in CSU. ©MB

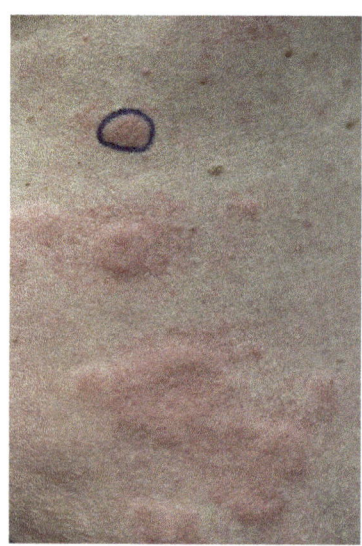

FIG. 2: Wheal marked with a pen to determine its duration. ©MB

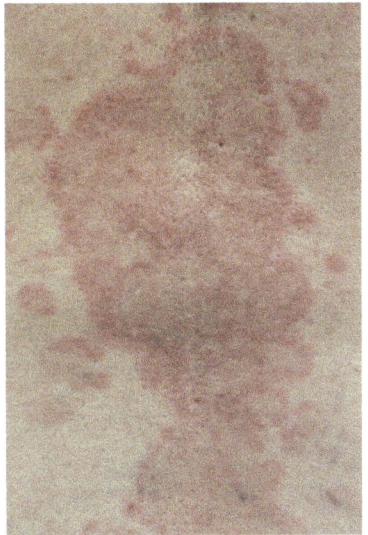

FIG. 3: Annular and polycyclic wheals in CSU. ©MB

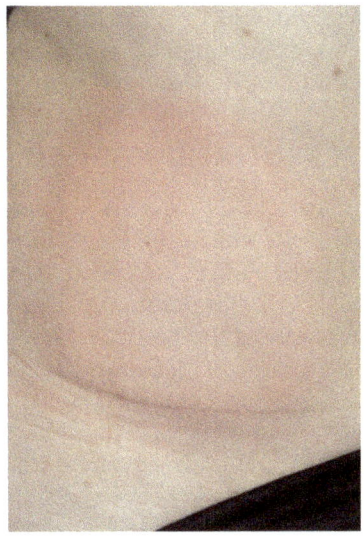

FIG. 4: Large wheal in CSU. ©MB

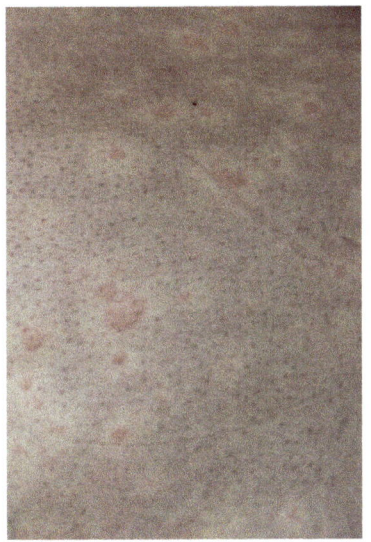

FIG. 5: Wheals surrounded by blanching. ©MB

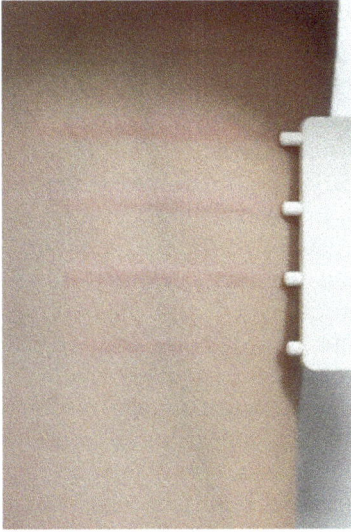

FIG. 6: Wheals in symptomatic dermographism shaped according to the trigger. ©MB

palm-sized lesions (**Figs. 1** to **5**). They are often surrounded by reflex erythema (**Figs. 1** and **2**) and rarely by blanching (**Fig. 5**). If lesions are not active at the time of examination, patients' own photographs can help establish the diagnosis. There are no clinical signs of epidermal damage, e.g., scale, crusting, and vesicles. Patients rub their wheals and excoriations are rare. Some forms of chronic inducible urticaria (CIndU) are characterized by a specific appearance of wheals, e.g., wheals confined to the site of friction in symptomatic dermographism (**Fig. 6**).

Angioedema is a transient, localized swelling of the deeper layers of the skin, e.g., lips, eyelids, hands, feet or mucosa, e.g., tongue. It is mostly nonpruritic, but can be painful. The lesions last longer, but just as wheals, they resolve completely.

DIFFERENTIAL DIAGNOSIS OF ACUTE URTICARIA

Acute urticaria presents as scattered wheals, at times accompanied by angioedema, that last <6 weeks but can recur. It is usally idiopathic, but it can also be triggered by an acute infection or drugs such as nonsteroidal anti-inflammatory drugs (NSAIDs) or antibiotics. Type I hypersensitivity [immunoglobulin E (IgE)-mediated allergy] to food may be relevant in selected cases. Food induced urticaria is usually shortlived (hours rather than days) and reproducible, e.g., patients allergic to a particular food react each time they consume it. Acute urticaria can occur in the context of *anaphylaxis,* in which exposure to an allergen, e.g., food, medications, and insect venom triggers the release of vasoactive mediators, often via an IgE-mediated pathway. Anaphylaxis is likely when there is an acute onset of generalized wheals and/or angioedema accompanied by respiratory symptoms, e.g., dyspnea, wheeze, and stridor; reduced blood pressure including syncope; gastrointestinal symptoms, e.g., abdominal pain and vomiting; symptoms from other systems, e.g., incontinence or uterine cramps.[2] Acute urticaria present for hours or days is not likely to evolve into anaphylaxis. *Maculopapular drug exanthem* is a T-cell mediated reaction that can occur within a few days to 2-3 weeks of the onset of almost any drug. There is usually a symmetrical eruption of itchy, confluent red macules, and papules that begin on the upper body and progesses distally to the extremities, persists for several days and is followed by desquamation. *Viral exanthem* may present as a macular, maculopapular, urticarial, and/or vesicular reaction that lasts a few days and may be associated with mucosal lesions, fever or other systemic symptoms. *Insect bites or stings* may cause urticarial skin lesions, which usually last >24 hours and may have a central hemorrhagic punctum, vesicle or crust. *Pityriasis rosea* is characterized by an eruption of sharply defined, round or oval pink macules or plaques, covered by fine (usually marginal) scales. They are mainly seen on the trunk. *Erythema multiforme* is an acute eruption of dull red, macular, papular or urticarial lesions often with "target appearance" with multiple concentric color zones. Lesions are preferentially distributed on distal extremities. They appear in successive crops for a few days, slowly enlarge, and fade in 1-2 weeks. *Sweet's syndrome (acute febrile neutrophilic dermatosis)* is characterized by fever and acute onset of painful, erythematous papules, plaques or nodules, often with a pseudovesicular aspect, that persist for days to weeks. *Polymorphic light eruption* usually occurs in spring. Symmetrically distributed itchy, erythematous skin lesions (mainly papules, plaques or vesicles) appear and persist for several days.[3]

DIFFERENTIAL DIAGNOSIS OF CHRONIC URTICARIA

Recurring wheals and/or angioedema are not specific for CU. They occur in other skin diseases which should be suspected in patients refractory to standard CU treatment or if itching is scarce and patients have other symptoms, e.g., arthralgia and fever.[1,4] *Urticarial vasculitis (UV)* is characterized by recurrent urticarial rashes with lesions that remain fixed at one site for >24 hours (even several days), and have histopathologic findings of leukocytoclastic vasculitis.[5] Skin lesions slowly change in size and shape, can be painful, and often resolve with bruising and/or postinflammatory hyperpigmentation (**Fig. 7**).[6] UV can also present with angioedema, purpura, and extracutaneous manifestations related to systemic vasculitis, e.g., arthralgia, lymphadenopathy, abdominal pain, ocular and renal manifestations as well as dyspnea/cough. The worldwide prevalence of UV is unknown.[5,7] It is usually idiopathic, but it can be associated with drugs, infections, malignancy, and autoimmunity.[5,6] Up to 20% of patients with systemic lupus erythematosus reportedly have UV.[8] The diagnosis is ultimately made with the histopathological evaluation of a lesional skin biopsy (**Fig. 7**).

Suggested laboratory studies include a full (complete) blood count, blood biochemistry, serum creatinine, C-reactive protein (CRP), erythrocyte sedimentation rate (ESR), urinalysis, complement studies (C1q, C3, C4), anti-C1q antibody assays, and tests for underlying connective tissue disease, e.g., antinuclear antibody (ANA), antineutrophil cytoplasmic antibodies (ANCA), rheumatoid factor or viral infection, e.g., hepatitis and human immunodeficiency virus (HIV). Based on complement level, UV is divided into normocomplementemic urticarial vasculitis (NUV), hypocomplementemic urticarial vasculitis (HUV) or hypocomplementemic urticarial vasculitis syndrome (HUVS).[7] About 80% of all UV patients have NUV[7] which can be difficult to distinguish clinically from severe forms of CSU, even on histopathology.[9,10] HUV and HUVS are the most severe forms of UV and are often associated with long duration and underlying disorders.[5] Anti-C1q antibodies were found in 55% of HUV patients, but they are not specific and may be observed in patients with primary and secondary vasculitis.[6] *Autoinflammatory diseases (AIDs)* are rare and severely debilitating chronic diseases that involve persistent history of recurrent urticarial lesions (rarely angioedema), neutrophilic leukocytosis, and elevated inflammation markers such as CRP, ESR, and serum amyloid A (SAA).[1,6,11] The rash usually consists of flat erythematous wheals lasting up to 24 hours, distributed on the trunk and/or extremities with head sparing. They do not respond to antihistamines. Pruritus may be absent but the lesions can be painful. AID are often diagnosed with a delay of years or even decades.[11] They may be hereditary or acquired. *Cryopyrin-associated periodic syndromes (CAPS)* are hereditary AID characterized by episodes of fever, urticaria-such as rash, fatigue, headaches, arthralgia, arthritis, myalgia, sensorineural hearing loss, ocular inflammation, and/or bone lesions. They often manifest in early childhood. Inflammation is caused by an inappropriate activation of the innate immunity and overproduction of the proinflammatory cytokine interleukin-1 (IL-1).[1,6] *Schnitzler syndrome* is an acquired AID that usually starts in the fifth decade of life. It is characterized by recurrent fever, urticaria-such as rash, arthralgia, arthritis, myalgia, lymphadenopathy, hepatosplenomegaly, and monoclonal gammopathy (IgM or less commonly IgG class). Its pathophysiology remains unclear, but it is assumed to be IL-1 mediated.[1,6,11,12] About 15% of patients develop a lymphoproliferative disorder.[11] Anti-IL1 drugs (e.g., anakinra) can effectively control AID, but if left untreated, chronic inflammation with continuously elevated SAA may cause amyloidosis.[6,11] If AID is suspected, testing for elevated inflammatory markers, serum protein electrophoresis to rule out monoclonal gammopathy in adults, urinalysis to screen for proteinuria due to secondary renal amyloidosis and skin

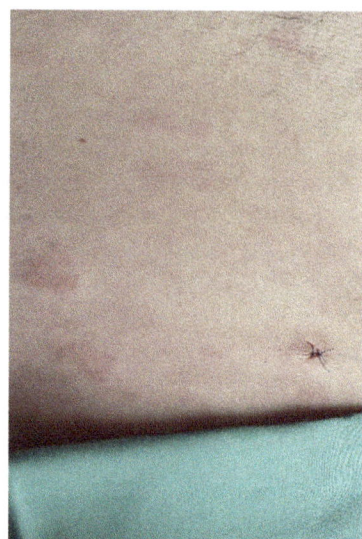

FIG. 7: Lesions of urticarial vasculitis resolving with bruising. ©MB

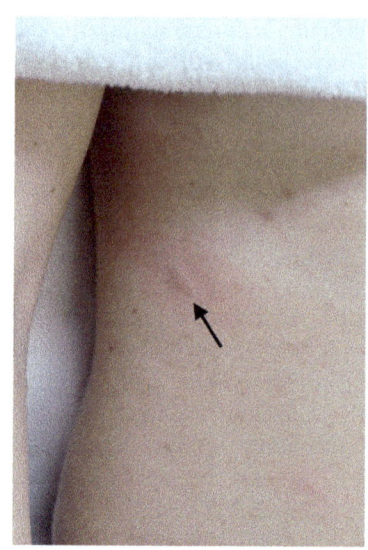

FIG. 8: Darier's sign in maculopapular cutaneous mastocytosis. ©MB

biopsy to look for neutrophil-rich infiltrates are indicated. If hereditary AID is suspected, testing for mutation in the relevant genes should also be considered. *Gleich syndrome (episodic angioedema with eosinophilia)* is characterized by cyclic episodes of angioedema, wheals, fever, characteristic weight gain, and dramatic eosinophilia.[13] *Maculopapular cutaneous mastocytosis* is characterized by multiple hyperpigmented macular or maculopapular lesions that urticate within a few minutes when rubbed or scratched (Darier's sign, **Fig. 8**).[14]

Bullous pemphigoid commonly starts with a nonspecific rash, with an occasionally urticarial appearance. It usually lasts 1–3 weeks before blisters develop, which may be similar to some urticarial dermatoses in pregnancy, e.g., *pemphigoid gestationis. Erythema annulare centrifugum* is characterized by solitary or multiple erythematous, ring-shaped, and polycyclic plaques that slowly spread peripherally and may show a characteristic slight scaling behind the advancing edge. *Autoimmune progesterone dermatitis* is triggered by hypersensitivity to progesterone. Variable skin lesions, e.g., resembling wheals or eczema recur cyclically in the premenstrual period.[3] *Urticarial dermatitis* occurs mostly in elderly patients and presents with highly pruritic eczematous and urticarial lesions, either simultaneously or sequentially. It is difficult to treat and may be idiopathic or represent the initial presentation of several skin diseases, namely bullous pemphigoid or drug eruptions.[15-17]

DIFFERENTIAL DIAGNOSIS OF ANGIOEDEMA WITHOUT WHEALS

Angioedema without wheals represents a distinct clinical pattern with several subtypes (**Box 1**).

> **Box 1: Recurrent angioedema without wheals.**
>
> *Mast cell-mediated angioedema*
> *Bradykinin-mediated angioedema*
> - Angiotensin-converting enzyme (ACE) inhibitor-associated angioedema
> - Hereditary angioedema with quantitative or functional C1 inhibitor deficiency
> - Hereditary angioedema without C1 inhibitor deficiency
> - Angioedema due to acquired C1 inhibitor deficiency
>
> *Angioedema of unknown cause*

Early diagnosis is essential since effective treatment depends on the mediator responsible for increased vascular permeability.[13,18] *Mast cell-mediated angioedema* is triggered by mast cell-mediators, including histamine. It responds well to antihistamines, glucocorticoids, and adrenaline (epinephrine). Around 10% of CSU patients have angioedema without wheals.[18] In CSU, it can last up to 72 hours[1] and commonly starts on the head or neck in the early morning hours.[18] Mast cell-mediated angioedema may also occur in acute urticaria or during anaphylaxis. There are also IgE-independent mechanisms of mast cell activation, caused by drugs such as vancomycin or fluoroquinolones via Mas-related G protein-coupled receptor X2 (MRGPRX2) or NSAIDs via alterations in arachidonic acid metabolism. *Bradykinin-mediated angioedema* is triggered by bradykinin that promotes vasodilatation and causes angioedema (but no wheals). It responds poorly to standard CU medications, lasts up to 3–5 days and may cause a dangerous swelling of the larynx and oropharynx.[4,18] *Angiotensin-converting enzyme (ACE) inhibitor-associated angioedema* is relatively common. It may occur months, or even years, after start of ACE inhibitor treatment. *Hereditary angioedema with quantitative or functional C1 inhibitor deficiency* is an autosomal dominant disorder caused by mutations in the C1 inhibitor (C1-INH) gene. C1-INH deficiency results in bradykinin overproduction. *Angioedema due to acquired C1-INH deficiency* is often accompanied by a lymphoproliferative or autoimmune disorder that leads to continuous activation of the classic complement pathway with consequent depletion of C1-INH. Any patient with:

- Recurrent angioedema without wheals nonresponsive to standard CU treatment and
- Not taking ACE inhibitors and
- Not experiencing remission after 6 months of ACE inhibitor avoidance should be screened for complement deficiency.

If C4 level is low, C1-INH quantification and function need to be determined. The underlying pathomechanism of some cases of recurrent angioedema without wheals remains unknown.[18] Angioedema also needs to be distinguished from other conditions characterized by swellings, especially when standard angioedema treatments fail to achieve desirable clinical outcomes. *Granulomatous cheilitis* is characterized by intermittent lip swelling in the initial stage, followed by persistent swelling of the lips, occasionally extending to the face due to granulomatous inflammation of unknown cause.[13] In *cellulitis* and *erysipelas* there is inflammation of dermal and subcutaneous tissue due to an infective trigger. Localized area of the body becomes bright red, swollen, painful, and hot. There are often systemic manifestations. *Wells syndrome (eosinophilic cellulitis)* presents with a swelling resembling cellulitis.[3] *Autoimmune hypothyroidism, dermatomyositis,* and *Sjögren's syndrome* may present with periorbital swelling resembling angioedema of the eyelids.[13] Diffuse swelling of the face and neck due to *superior vena cava syndrome* may also mimic angioedema. *Allergic contact dermatitis* may be misdiagnosed as facial angioedema. Initial clinical differentiation from angioedema may be challenging, but the swelling in contact dermatitis slowly spreads in direction of gravity and eventually resolves. Clinical signs reflecting changes of the epidermis, i.e., erythema, vesicles, scale, and crusting also appear and regress faster if treated with glucocorticoids. Patch testing is required to confirm hypersensitivity.

 ONLINE REFERENCES

To access the references of this chapter online, kindly refer to **emedicine360.com** also please follow the instructions mentioned on inside cover.

CHAPTER 10

Diagnostic Approach

Maryam Al-Nesf, Riccardo Asero,
L Karla Arruda

URTICARIA DIAGNOSTIC APPROACH

INTRODUCTION

Urticaria is a challenging disease to manage and control. It causes a burden not only on the affected individuals and their quality of life but also on the treating physician and the health system. In particular, chronic urticaria (CU) brings emotional burden. Also, the patients' expectations in most instances cannot be accommodated by the currently available medical regimen and the guidance to resolve and back to normal is limited.[1] Acute urticaria usually requires no much diagnostic workup. In most instances, it is benign and self-limited with mainly symptomatic treatment by using oral antihistamines, although patients experiencing severe and abrupt acute urticaria may ask for assistance at the emergency departments where they are invariably treated with injection corticosteroids and antihistamines. If the acute urticaria has clinical features suggesting it may progress into a chronic illness, such patients should be periodically re-evaluated until the disease is resolved or a diagnosis is clarified.[2] However, acute urticaria can signify underlying more severe and serious diseases, including anaphylaxis.[3] Moreover, if the recurrent lesions were just isolated angioedema without urticaria, the treating physician should consider hereditary angioedema and drug-induced, such as angiotensin-converting enzyme (ACE)-inhibitors-induced angioedema.

On the other hand, CU mandates a comprehensive medical history that, by itself, most of the time, is sufficient to establish the correct diagnosis and the exact type and exclude other medical conditions mimicking urticaria.[4] A systematic approach with a stepwise selection of the appropriate diagnostic technique is required to diagnose urticaria correctly. Multiple approaches and guidelines were used to diagnose urticaria. A personalized approach using a step-by-step approach was evaluated.[5] An easy-to-use checklist was used to facilitate medical history taking and evaluate the disease control and burden.[6] Using a multidisciplinary approach[7] and taking a comprehensive history[4-6] continue to be key elements to be incorporated in the diagnosis and management of CU.

Perera E et al. utilized a simple diagnostic approach that is important for busy primary care practitioner clinics to identify the urticaria subtypes and the patients' clinical needs, leading to the appropriate management,[4] while Cherrez–Ojeda et al. used a customized checklist based on patient medical history to identify the different types.[6]

This review aims to focus on a personalized diagnostic approach based on the previously used approaches, checklist, and international CU guidelines.[2,4-6,8] Three key elements are important for the diagnostic approach of CU. The first one is to confirm the correct diagnosis of acute versus chronic, exclude other differential diagnoses, and reach the correct classification of either chronic spontaneous urticaria (CSU) (previously called idiopathic) or chronic induced urticaria (CINDU). The second is to determine the culprit or trigger. The third is to assess the urticaria activity scoring, degree of control, and impact on life.[4,8]

In the diagnostic approach of urticaria, the first step is to take a detailed and systemic anamnesis and perform a comprehensive physical examination to promptly evaluate the clinical presentation of patients attending with CU, aiming to gather all possible provoking factors and causes of CU. Important questions to include are the duration of urticaria (less or more than 6 weeks), frequency and duration of hive lesions (less or more than 24 hours), and the presence of diurnal variation. The size, shape, color, and distribution of the lesions should be collected. The associated subjective symptoms of the lesion (erythema, wheals, edema, pruritus, burning, or itching) are of significant guidance to assess the burden of the disease and how far the quality of life is affected. These symptoms should be revisited while on a different regimen of treatments until control is achieved. Using a scoring system that will be discussed later provides guidance for the patient and the physicians of the disease severity and control. Other descriptions of the lesions (pruritus, burning, pain, or blistering) and other features that may accompany the urticaria like syndromes (e.g., petechia, ecchymosis, Raynaud phenomena, livedo reticularis, and postlesion hyperpigmentation) should be gathered. If the hives are accompanied by angioedema, a detailed angioedema description should be evaluated, including the triggering factor and the angioedema characteristic if localized or generalized. Apart from subcutaneous angioedema, mucosal edema involving the respiratory, throat, and digestive tracts may be hidden findings and should be sought by direct questions of these systems when taking a detailed history and examination. In particular, the physician should ask about wheezing (respiratory), change in voice or throat closure (throat), and abdominal pain and vomiting (gastroenterology). Involvement of other organs and systems, such as joints, eyes, kidneys, neurology, and symptoms of systematic involvement (fever, joint pain, weight loss, or malaise) should be noted. Previous or currently existing allergies, infections, other medical diseases, or other possible causes and family history regarding urticaria like atopy or other immunological diseases should always be part of the urticaria anamnesis to guide in excluding other differentials. Medication history including intake of nonsteroidal anti-inflammatory drugs (NSAIDs), injections, immunizations, hormones, laxatives, and alternative remedies) as well as food; smoking habits; type of work; hobbies; occurrence in relation to weekends, holidays, and foreign travel; surgical implantations; reactions to insect stings; relationship to the menstrual cycle; response to therapy; and stress; all should be taken.[9]

The second step is to search for the triggering culprit of the wheals and angioedema by conducting specific provocation testing based on the collected medical history. At this stage, the physician is able to distinguish between CSU from CINDU and determine the individual trigger thresholds.[10] Physical urticaria is one subtype of CINDU. It has many names depending on the cause and the test used to confirm the diagnosis. Examples are cold (where an ice cube is left in contact with the skin of the forearm for 5 minutes), heat (heat stimulus using a test tube with water >44° or a heated cylinder), vibration (a vibrating instrument like a vortex), sun [photo-test by differing levels of ultraviolet A (UVA) and UVB radiation on 1 cm sections of the skin], or pressure.[6] Stroking the skin with a blunt, firm object such as tongue depressor or a calibrated instrument, like a dermographometer (HTZ, Croydon, UK) or FricTest (Moxie, Berlin, and Germany), usually on the upper back or across the skin of the patient arm is a simple test to elicit wheals and flare and confirm the diagnosis of dermographism.[11] In contrast, delayed pressure urticaria is confirmed by applying pressure of 0.2–0.4 kg/cm^2 for 10 and 20 minutes.[6] Other nonphysical forms of CINDU should always be considered, such as cholinergic urticaria (exercise, with or without hot bath and sweating) and aquagenic urticaria (applying for 20 minutes a piece of cloth impregnated in body temperature water).[9] Contact (work-related) urticaria is another form that may be underestimated in the clinical practice and can be triggered by skin contact with wheal/angioedema-inducing substances. In the UK, its rate is estimated to be 3–4 per million population.[12] A big list of agents was attributed to induce occupational contact urticaria (OCU); the most common are natural rubber latex and sorbic acid.[13] A significant decline in OCU is due to a reduction in the use of natural rubber latex among health care workers in Europe.[12,14] Other reported work-related triggers should always be considered according to each patient's job. Evaluating if the symptoms improved or even disappeared during weekends and holidays and type of work is crucial in taking a medical history.[13] Some patients may exhibit more than one physical type or unable to describe the potential trigger appropriately, for which we recommend testing more than one or even all until confirming the triggering factors. Moreover, two or more concurrent triggers may be needed to produce an urticarial rash in rare patients. It is important to give enough time for the hive to develop and have a good time of observation in the clinic as patients may develop other than skin manifestations of the disease during the provocation test, and this may range from other system involvement (dizziness, wheezing or vomiting) to full-blown anaphylaxis. For this reason, such tests should be performed by physicians trained and experienced in the emergency treatment of allergic responses and where facilities for emergency treatment are available, including the use of adrenaline and possible intubation.[10] So, risk stratification should always be examined before conducting tests in the clinic based on the patients' medical history and reviewing his medical record and medical notes of emergency visits. In patients with a very high-risk of developing anaphylaxis, the extreme of age, or multiple comorbidities, such tests may be carried out under more controlled settings like in the hospital inpatient or short-stay services. Other provoking factors that must be included are insects with excluding insects-induced anaphylaxis and cellulitis (Skeeters syndrome), infections, food, drugs, tobacco use, and in female patients, the state resulted in hormonal changes such as pregnancy and menstrual cycles. Stress is a very well-known immunologically provoking factor. Urticaria and several psychological or psychiatric disorders may be interconnected, among which sleep-wake, anxiety, trauma and stressor-related, somatic symptom, obsessive-compulsive, substance-related and addictive, and mood disorders were evaluated and significantly associated with the diagnosis of urticaria.[7]

Laboratory work has a very limited role to help in the diagnostic approach. Complete blood count with differentials, C-reactive protein (CRP), thyroid function test, liver and kidney functions, complements (C3, C4, C1q, and CH50), and ruling out infections including *Helicobacter pylori*, acute hepatitis, and other viruses such as cytomegalovirus (CMV) and Epstein–Barr virus (EBV) are among the most relevant tests. Food and drug allergies are evaluated by total and specific immunoglobulin E (IgE) (skin prick test or blood test and/or skin patch test) for the expected food or drug when available or through challenges. Autoantibodies, mast cell tryptase, should not be routinely done unless other differentials are suspected or the patient shows a poor response to treatment. An autologous serum/plasma skin test (ASST) is an easy test to perform in the clinic, may help to confirm the diagnosis of autoreactive CSU. A skin biopsy should be done by a qualified expert and preserved for cases where the clinical picture and skin lesions are not agreeable with CSU and CINDU and not usual for other common dermatology conditions (**Flowchart 1**).[6]

The final step in the diagnostic approach is to evaluate disease activity and severity, degree of control, and the impact on life. Multiple scoring systems exist that can help in evaluating the disease severity and response to treatment. Urticaria Activity Score in 7 days (UAS7) provides semi-quantitative information on disease activity between clinic visits and captures changes in intensity and possible triggers. Angioedema Activity Score (AAS) is a tool that assesses angioedema activity; however, it provides an incomplete component score of angioedema, hives, and itch. The utilization of the Urticaria Control Test (UCT) is allowing to assess

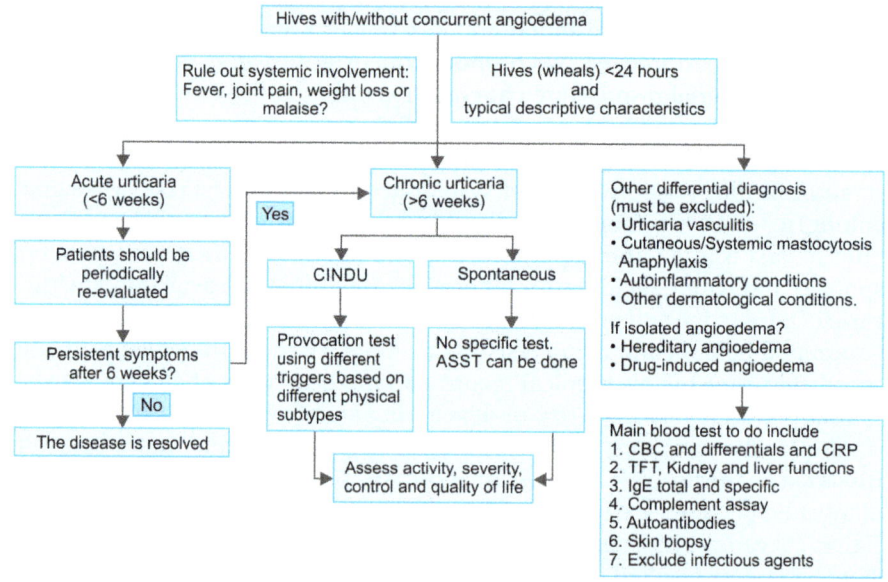

(ASST: autologous serum/plasma skin test; CINDU: chronic inducible urticaria; CBC: complete blood count; CRP: C-reactive protein; TFT: thyroid function test; IgE: immunoglobulin E)

FLOWCHART 1: Diagnostic approach for patients with urticaria.

Source: Adapted from references 2–6 and 8–10.

disease control over the past 4 weeks. The final scoring instruments are Chronic Urticaria Quality of Life Questionnaire (CU-Q2oL), focusing on within six domains: Functioning, sleep, itching/embarrassment/mental status, swelling/eating, limits, and looks and the AngioEdema (AE-QoL) examining four dimensions: Functioning, fatigue/mood, fears/shame, and nutrition. Both questionnaires are used to evaluate the impact of the disease on the quality of affected individual life.

In summary, the patient history in diagnosis and assessment of disease severity and limited laboratory testing can confirm the diagnosis of CU and exclude underlying systemic diseases. Extended diagnostic testing may be used in some patients, particularly in CINDU, to identify thresholds of eliciting factors. Many validated scoring systems and assessment tools are available to help in the care of CU before and during the management course and to stratify disease severity, control, and impact on life.[5]

 ONLINE REFERENCES

To access the references of this chapter online, kindly refer to **emedicine360.com** also please follow the instructions mentioned on inside cover.

CHAPTER 11

Patient-reported Outcome Measures

Alicja Kasperska-Zajac, Solange Oliveira Rodrigues Valle, Sergio Duarte Dortas Junior, Agnieszka Sikora, Magdalena Zając, Maria Luiza Oliva Alonso

INTRODUCTION

Currently, there are no reliable biomarkers to identify and measure disease activity in chronic spontaneous urticaria (CSU). Consequently, the use of patient-reported outcomes (PROs) everyday medical practice is very useful and enables optimal management of this difficult disease, taking into account the patient's perception of their own disease and adapting the treatment to their needs.

The Urticaria Activity Score (UAS), the urticaria control test (UCT), and the chronic urticaria quality life questionnaire (CU-QO2L) are recommended by the European Academy of Allergology and Clinical Immunology/Global Allergy and Asthma European Network/European Dermatology Forum/World Allergy Organization (EAACI/GA2LEN/EDF/WAO) for standard management of urticaria.[1]

URTICARIA ACTIVITY SCORE

Overall description: UAS is a PROs tool to measure disease activity in CSU.[1-3]

Purpose: To assess CSU activity/severity and treatment response.[3,4]

Method of administration/recall period: Patient-reported prospective assessments; diary-type tool documented everyday for 7 days (UAS7).[1,3-4]

Number of items/content: Two components; number of wheals (ranging from 0: none to 3: >50 wheals) and intensity of itch (ranging from 0: none to 3: severe).[3,4] Patients are asked to document in 24-hour intervals, and the summed result gives a daily UAS score (0–6 points). Due to the unpredictability of wheals and itching, it is recommended that UAS should be done for 7 consecutive days, to compensate for fluctuations that commonly occur in disease activity.[5,6]

Response option/scoring/score interpretation: This score is summed over 7 days before medical visit, giving the UAS7 score (0–42 points).[3-6] Cut-off values have been proposed as follows: A UAS7 score of 7–15 indicates mild disease activity, a UAS7 score of 16–27 indicates moderate disease activity, and a UAS7 score of 28–42 indicates severe disease activity.[7]

Patient burden/administrative burden: The instrument takes <1 minute to complete; time to score minimal.[5,6]

Minimal clinical important difference (MCID): 11 points for UAS7.[8]

Translations/Adaptations: The original German version has been translated and validated in multiple languages.[3,4]

Clinical and research usability: Routine practice and trials/studies.

It is important to note that the UAS7 is only applicable to CSU and not suitable for chronic inducible urticaria (CIndU). However, CIndU-specific activity scores are available (CholUAS7 for cholinergic urticaria) or in development (ColdUAS for cold urticaria, SDAS for symptomatic dermographism).[9]

URTICARIA CONTROL TEST

Overall description: The UCT was developed specifically to assess the control status and therapeutic response, complementing the shortcomings of UAS7. To determine the level of disease control in all forms of chronic urticaria (CU): CSU (with or without angioedema), CIndU, and combinations of both subtypes.[4,10]

Purpose: To determine the level of disease control in all forms of CU: CSU (with or without angioedema), CIndU, and combinations of both subtypes.[4,10]

Number of items/content: Originally developed two forms: The long form UCT (UCTlg) (8 questions) and the short form UCT (UCTsh) (4 questions).[4,10,11]

Method of administration/recall period: Patient self-report retrospective questionnaire; recall period of 4 weeks; it is performed and assessed during a patient consultation.[4,10,11]

Response option/scoring/score interpretation: Five answer options for each of the 4 items that are scored from 0 to 4 points; the range of summary score is 0–16, where a higher value indicates a higher level of urticaria control, a cut off of 12 is used to identify patients with "well-controlled," and "poorly controlled" (<12 points) urticaria.[10,11]

Patient burden/administrative burden: The time to complete is very short (<1 minute), simple, and quick for hand-scoring.[10]

Reliability/Validity: Internal consistency reliability is excellent, and level of convergent validity is high.[10,11]

MCID: 3 points for UCTsh.[12]

Origin/Development/Translation/Adaptation: This test was developed and validated by a team led by Dr Karsten Weller and Dr Marcus Maurer in German and American English. The version is still being translated and validated in different languages.

Clinical and research usability: Suitable for use in routine practice and studies in the adult population. An ideal way is to use both UAS7 and UCT in CU patients, as they would allow the physician to better understand disease activity as well as to assess disease control and therapeutic response.[1,3]

Availability: Moxie GmbH (www.moxie-gmbh.de).

CHRONIC URTICARIA QUALITY LIFE QUESTIONNAIRE

Overall description: The CU-Q2oL was developed specifically to assess the impact of CU on quality of life in patients with CSU.[1,3,13,14]

Purpose: To assess the impact of CU on health-related quality of life from the patient's perspective.[14]

Method of administration/recall period: Self-administered questionnaire covering the previous 2 weeks; it is performed right before or during a patient consultation.[4,13]

Number of items/content: The questionnaire has 23 items divided into six domains: Pruritus (2 items), edema (2 items), impact on daily activities (6 items), impact on sleep (5 items), limitations (3 items), and physical appearance (5 items), according to the validation study of the original version.[14]

In Brazilian version, the items are divided into three domains: (1) sleep/mental state/food, (2) pruritus/impact of activities, and (3) edema/limitations/appearance.[15]

Response option/scoring/score interpretation: A five-point Likert scale the intensity of each item separately (ranging from 0: "nothing" to 5: "very much"). For each of the six dimensions a score is calculated, and then a total index for all dimensions. Minimum total score is 23. Higher values reflect greater impairment of the symptom-specific health-related QoL. The score can be converted to a scale of 0–100 to facilitate comparisons with other questionnaires.[14,15]

MCID: 15 points for CU-Q2oL was proposed in the Thai study.[16]

Patient burden/administrative burden: The questionnaire takes <5 minutes to complete; easy scoring if quick assessment forms are available (e.g., online calculator and scoring template).

Translations/adaptations: This test was developed and validated by a team led by Dr Baiardini in Italy. The original Italian version has been translated and validated in multiple languages.[15-17]

Clinical and research usability: Routine practice and trials/studies. It should be applied at least every 6 months.

It is important to note that the CU-Q2oL has some limitations: It is only applicable to CSU and not suitable for CIndU, validated for adults only, lack of categorization of severity and more specific questions about the impact of angioedema.

PROs in Recurrent Angioedema

The Angioedema Quality of Life Questionnaire (AE-QoL), the Angioedema Activity Score (AAS), and the Angioedema Control Test (AECT) are recommended by EAACI/GA2LEN/EDF/WAO for standard management of angioedema.[1]

Angioedema Quality of Life Questionnaire

Overall description: AE-QoL is the first validated disease-specific instrument for assessment of QoL impairment in patients with predominant angioedema (with or without wheals).[1,18]

Purpose: To measure the impact of angioedema on health-related QoL from the patient's perspective.[1,18]

Method of administration/recall period: Self-administered questionnaire covering the previous 4 weeks.[18]

Number of QoL items/domain: The instrument includes 17 items which cover 4 domains related to the impact of angioedema on functioning, fatigue/mood, fear/shame, and food.[18]

Response option/scoring/score interpretation: Each item has 5 answer options. The total score is transformed into a linear scale from 0 to 100, with higher values reflecting greater impairment of the symptom-specific health-related QoL.[18] According to the Thai version of AE-QoL, total values of 0–23, 24–38, and ≥ 39 could classify patients into 3 groups: "no effect", "small effect", and "moderate to large effect" of their disease on QoL.[19]

MCID: A change in AE-QoL >6 points is interpreted as the smallest difference in score that reflects a meaningful improvement in the symptom-specific health-related QoL.[20]

Patient burden/administrative burden: The questionnaire takes <5 minutes to complete; easy scoring if quick assessment forms are available (e.g., online calculator and scoring template).

Translations/Adaptations: The original German version of AE-QoL has been translated and validated in multiple languages.[1]

Clinical and research usability: Routine practice and clinical trials/studies in adults.

Multilanguage availability: Moxie GmbH (www.moxie-gmbh.de).

Angioedema Activity Score

Overall description: AAS is the first validated PROs tool to measure disease activity in angioedema.[21]

Purpose: To assess and monitor disease activity in adult patients with predominant angioedema (with or without wheals).[1,21,22]

Method of administration/recall period: Patient-reported prospective assessments; diary-type tool documented everyday for 4 weeks (AAS28).[21]

Number of items/content: Five question; the main question is whether the angioedema has occurred in the last 24 hours. If the answer is yes, five additional questions are asked about "severity of physical discomfort caused by angioedema", "ability to perform daily activities during presence of angioedema", "cosmetic disfigurement caused by angioedema" and" global assessment of impairment, and severity caused by angioedema", which refer to the 8-hour period after the onset of angioedema.[21]

Response option/scoring/score interpretation: Four answer options for each of the 5 items ranging from 0 (none) to 3 (severe); the range for cumulative daily AAS score is 0–15, the weekly AAS (AAS7) is 0–105, and monthly AAS (AAS28) is 0–420, where a higher value indicates a higher level of angioedema activity/severity.[21]

Patient burden/administrative burden: The instrument takes <1 minute to complete; time to score minimal.

MCID: 8 points for AAS7.[21]

Translations/Adaptations: The original German version has been translated and validated in multiple languages.

Clinical and research usability: Routine practice and trials/studies.

Multilanguage availability: Moxie GmbH (www.moxie-gmbh.de).

Angioedema Control Test

Overall description: The AECT is a novel tool for assessing disease control and making therapeutic decisions in patients with recurrent angioedema of various subtypes, including hereditary angioedema and acquired angioedema due to C1-inhibitor deficiency, CSU-associated angioedema, and idiopathic angioedema.[23,24]

Purpose: To measure the level of disease control from the perspective of patients with predominant angioedema (with or without wheals).[23,24]

Number of items/content: Four simple questions about "How often have you had angioedema?", "How much has your quality of life been affected by angioedema?", "How much has the unpredictability of your angioedema bothered you?", and "How well has your angioedema been controlled by your therapy?".[23,24]

Method of administration/recall period: Patient self-report retrospective questionnaire; two versions available with a recall period of 4 weeks (AECT-4 weeks) or 3 months (AECT-3 months); it is performed and assessed during a patient consultation.[23,24]

Response option/scoring/score interpretation: Five answer options for each of the 4 items that are scored from 0 to 4 points; the range of summary score is 0–16, where a higher value indicates a higher level of angioedema control; a cut off of 10 is used to identify patients with "well-controlled" and "poorly controlled" (<10 points) angioedema.[23,24]

Patient burden/administrative burden: The time to complete is very short (<1 minute); simple and quick for hand-scoring.

Reliability/Validity: Internal consistency reliability is excellent and level of convergent validity is high.

MCID: Not established.

Origin/Development/Translation/Adaptation: Like AE-QoL and AAS, this test was developed and validated by a team led by Dr Karsten Weller and Dr Marcus Maurer in German and American English.[23,24] The version is still being translated and validated in different languages.

Clinical and research usability: Suitable for use in routine practice and studies in the adult population.

Availability: Moxie GmbH (www.moxie-gmbh.de).

 ONLINE REFERENCES

To access the references of this chapter online, kindly refer to **emedicine360.com** also please follow the instructions mentioned on inside cover.

CHAPTER 12

Antihistamines

Anant Patil, Gordon Sussman, Nidhi Sharma

INTRODUCTION

Histamine is one of the most well studied chemicals having important physiological actions in human body.[1] It is one of the important mediators involved in the pathophysiology of allergic conditions.[2] The actions of histamine are mediated through H_1 receptors present on endothelial cells and sensory nerves. Action on endothelial cells results in wheals whereas actions on sensory nerve produce neurogenic flare and pruritus.[3] The histamine receptor is a member of G-protein coupled receptors.[1,4] The effects of histamine are governed by actions on four receptors named as H_1, H_2, H_3, and H_4.[1,2,5,6]

ANTIHISTAMINES

Antihistamines are not structurally related to histamines. They do not antagonize the binding of histamine to the receptor. Instead, they bind to the different place on the receptor resulting in opposite effect.[4] They act on histamine H_1 receptor and stabilize the inactive conformation of the receptor. This results in interference with actions of histamine H_1 receptors.[7] Considering this, these agents are not antagonists, but are inverse agonists.[4,7] The preferred term, thus is H_1-antihistamines.[4] H_1-antihistamines and H_2-antihistamines play an important role in the management of allergic conditions and gastrointestinal disorders respectively.[1]

Classification of Antihistamines

Based on the era of their development antihistamines are broadly classified into two types; first generation and second generation. The earlier drugs introduced in the market are known as first generation antihistamines. **Table 1** enlists examples of first generation and second generation antihistamine.[3,6]

Limitations of Older First Generation Antihistamines

Older first generation antihistamines are associated with following limitations:[3,5,7,8]
- First generation H_1-antihistamines have poor receptor selectivity and hence often interact with other receptors resulting in anticholinergic effects (urinary retention, tachycardia, thirst, etc.), antialpha adrenergic, and antiserotoninergic effects.

TABLE 1: Classification of first and second generation antihistamines.	
First generation antihistamines	**Second generation antihistamines**
• Chlorpheniramine maleate • Hydroxyzine • Promethazine • Diphenhydramine • Doxepin	• Cetirizine • Desloratadine • Fexofenadine • Levocetirizine • Acrivastine • Ebastine • Mizolastine • Bilastine • Rupatadine

- Brain H_1 receptor occupation is up to 80%, hence cause sedation
- Duration of action and antipruritic effect of first generation H_1-antihistamines is short (about 4–6 hours).
- First generation H_1-antihistamines are associated with interactions with several drugs (e.g., alcohol, medicines acting on central nervous system, and monoamine oxidase inhibitors).
- They interfere with rapid eye movement (REM) sleep. This results in cognitive and psychomotor impairment. This may result in impairment at school and driving performance.
- These agents also have potential for negative effect on learning and performance (work efficiency).
- They can lead to potentially life-threatening toxicity when taken in overdose.
- They have cardiac toxicity which was unrecognized when they were brought to market in the 1940's and 1950's.
- First generation antihistamines are on the Beers list of potentially inappropriate medications for older people.

Classification of Antihistamines According to Sedation Potential

Based on the occupancy of H_1 receptors in the brain, antihistamines can be classified as nonsedating (<20% occupancy), less-sedating (20–50% occupancy), and sedating (>50% occupancy) antihistamines.[5] The examples of antihistamines based on sedative potential are given in **Table 2**.[5,9]

Among the group of nonsedating agents, fexofenadine and bilastine are classified as nonbrain penetrating antihistamines.[5]

PHARMACOKINETICS OF H_1-ANTIHISTAMINES

Absorption

After administration by the oral route, H_1-antihistamines are generally well absorbed. Peak plasma concentrations are achieved within 1–3 hours after administration in fasting subjects. Organic anion transport protein and P-glycoprotein can affect bioavailability of some antihistamines. Inducers of

TABLE 2: Classification of H_1-antihistamines based on sedative potential.		
Nonsedating H_1-antihistamines	Less-sedating H_1-antihistamines	Sedating H_1-antihistamines
• Bilastine 20 mg • Fexofenadine 60–120 mg • Levocetirizine 5 mg • Epinastine 20 mg • Ebastine 10 mg • Loratadine 10 mg • Terfenadine 60 mg • Cetirizine 10 mg • Olopatadine 5 mg • Bepotastine 10 mg • Rupatadine 10–20 mg	• Azelastine 1 mg • Mequitazine 3 mg • Cetirizine 20 mg	• d-chlorpheniramine 2 mg • Diphenhydramine 30 mg • Hydroxyzine 20 mg • Ketotifen 1 mg

P-glycoprotein (e.g., rifampin) may reduce absorption of fexofenadine whereas P-glycoprotein inhibitors (e.g., erythromycin and ketoconazole) may increase its absorption. P-glycoprotein reduces absorption of fexofenadine into the brain and other organs.[10]

Fexofenadine should not be taken with grapefruit juice. Similarly, absorption of bilastine is reduced by concomitant intake of grapefruit juice. Absorption of bilastine is affected by food hence it is advised for optimal absorption it should be taken on empty stomach.[5]

Antihistamines which are metabolized in the liver by the cytochrome p450 pathway may interact with other drugs which are similarly metabolized. These drug-drug interactions resulted in cardiac toxicity due to prolongation of the QT interval with terfenadine and astemizole being withdrawn from the market.[2]

Administration of aluminum/magnesium-containing antacids within 15 minutes of a fexofenadine can reduce its absorption. This mechanism is different than discussed before.[10]

Distribution

Plasma protein binding depends on the affinity of the drug to the plasma proteins. Higher plasma protein means lower fraction of pharmacologically active drug is available for systemic effects. H_1-antihistamines have differences in the plasma protein binding from 50 to 98%.[10] The peak concentration is achieved quickly after oral dose. Significant effect on skin may be seen within 30 minutes to 3 hours. The peak effect on the histamine-induced wheal and flare is generally seen after 4–8 hours of oral dose.[10]

Metabolism and Elimination

In patients with liver or renal impairment dose or frequency of administration may be necessary for some agents (**Table 3**).

Considering their long duration of action, most of the second generation antihistamines can be given as once daily dose.[10]

TABLE 3: Use of second generation antihistamines in kidney and liver impairment.

	Kidney impairment	Liver impairment
Bilastine	Dose adjustment is not necessary, but concomitant administration with P-gp inhibitors in moderate or serious failure should be avoided	In liver impairment it is not expected to increase systemic exposure higher than safety limits
Loratadine	Lower dose (10 mg every other day) is recommended in patients with renal insufficiency (GFR <30 mL/min)	Lower dose (10 mg every other day) is recommended in patients with liver impairment
Desloratadine	Dosage adjustment in patients with renal impairment is recommended	Dosage adjustment is recommended
Cetirizine	Dosing adjustment is required in moderate or severe impairment and patients on dialysis	Dosing adjustment may be necessary
Levocetirizine	• The dose should be reduced in mild impairment while dose and frequency should be reduced in moderate or severe renal impairment • Avoided in end-stage renal disease (CLcr <10 mL/min) and patients undergoing hemodialysis	No dose adjustment is required in only hepatic impairment. In both hepatic and renal impairment, dose adjustment is recommended
Fexofenadine	Recommended starting dose is 60 mg OD in adults and 30 mg OD in children with impaired renal function	Dose adjustment is not required
Ebastine	Dose adjustment not required	Dose adjustment is not required in mild-to-moderate impairment. In serious impairment >10 mg should not be administered

(GFR: glomerular filtration rate; GP: glycoprotein)

Advantages of Second Generation Antihistamines[3]
- These drugs are nonsedating/minimally sedating.
- They are generally nonimpairing and do not potentiate alcohol or sedatives. Driving ability and thought processing is generally not adversely affected.
- Efficacy of these drugs is as good or higher than first generation antihistamines.
- Duration of action is also longer.

Second-generation antihistamines including fexofenadine, mizolastine, ebastine, cetirizine, levocetirizine, loratadine, desloratadine, and azelastine are not associated with clinically significant cardiac effects or QT prolongation.[4]

Broadly, these agents can be classified as having amino group or carboxy groups. Those with amino group (loratadine and desloratadine) show anticholinergic activity whereas, those with carboxy group (bilastine, fexofenadine, cetirizine, levocetirizine, and ebastine) are devoid of this activity.[5]

Selection of H_1-antihistamine

Several factors including efficacy, sedative potential, safety, lifestyle of patients, comorbidities, other medications, and cost of therapy are considered while selecting one agent over the others.[11] Not all the drugs from the class of second-generation antihistamines are nonsedating or less-sedating.[5] Considering good safety profile, second generation nonsedating antihistamines are recommended for use as the first line symptomatic treatment for urticaria and allergic rhinitis. Loss of effectiveness of peripheral H_1-receptor activity with regular daily administration is not a concern.[10]

Off label use of sedating H_1-antihistamines as sleep-promoting agents should be avoided, as they adversely affect the quality of sleep. Residual effect may also be seen on the next day.[5] A systematic review of randomized controlled trials of H_1-antihistamines in chronic spontaneous urticaria suggested that several antihistamines are effective at standard doses of treatment. However, no single H_1-antihistamine is recognized as the most effective.[12]

Guideline Recommendations for the use of Antihistamines in Urticaria

Nonsedating antihistamines are recommended as first line treatment for the treatment of chronic urticaria. In patients not responding to the regular dose, it may be increased up to four times.[3] Continuous treatment with H_1-antihistamines is important in the treatment of chronic urticaria.[13] In patients with urticaria, routine use of old sedating first generation antihistamines is not recommended.[3]

In some patients, combination of nonsedating H_1-antihistamine with H_2-antihistamine may be useful, but the evidence for such therapy is lacking.[3]

Nonsedating second generation antihistamines are also recommended for the treatment of acute spontaneous urticaria.[3]

SUMMARY

First generation antihistamines are associated with several adverse effects mainly because of their poor receptor selectivity and penetration of blood brain barrier. Second generation antihistamines offer advantages over them, hence are recommended as first line therapy for treatment of chronic urticaria. Guidelines for the treatment of chronic urticaria recommend staring with standard dose of second generation, nonsedating antihistamine. In patients with inadequate/satisfactory response, dose can be increased up to four-fold. Well-designed clinical trials comparing safety and efficacy of different modern second generation antihistamines in patients with urticaria are required.

 ONLINE REFERENCES

To access the references of this chapter online, kindly refer to **emedicine360.com** also please follow the instructions mentioned on inside cover.

CHAPTER 13

Cyclosporine A

Aslı Gelincik, Semra Demir, Silvia Ferrucci

STRUCTURE, MECHANISM OF ACTION, AND COMMERCIALLY AVAILABLE FORMS

Cyclosporine A (CSA) is a lipophilic polypeptide derived from a fungi called *Tolypocladium inflatum*. CSA has been discovered at 70s as an antifungal agent. Later on, its immunosuppressive effect has been detected. CSA forms a complex by binding a protein called cyclophilin and this complex competitively inhibits calcineurin phosphatase which in turn leads to selective suppression of T cell activation by decreasing the production of cytokines such as interleukin-2 (IL-2), IL-3, IL-4, interferon-gamma (IFN-γ), tumor necrosis factor-alpha (TNF-α), and macrophage colony stimulating factors.[1] It can also moderately decrease mast cell mediator release.[2,3]

There are commercially available topical, oral, and parenteral CSA formulations. Depending on its metabolism, there are two commercially available oral CSA. The first is a nonmodified formula (Sandimmune®) which is metabolized by the enterohepatic pathway while the latter is a modified formula (Neoral®) with a higher bioavailability independent from enterohepatic circulation. In clinical practice, it is important for clinicians to continue with the initial brand and do not use these brands interchangeably if the patient's symptoms are controlled since they are not bioequivalent.[4]

INDICATIONS

Cyclosporine A is primarily used to treat organ transplant rejection for >40 years. Also, it is used in graft versus host disease, rheumatoid arthritis, psoriasis, atopic dermatitis, amyotrophic lateral sclerosis, nephrotic syndrome, and refractory uveitis.[5] After late 90s, it has been off-labelly used in chronic spontaneous urticaria (CSU).[2]

CYCLOSPORINE A IN CHRONIC URTICARIA

In clinical trials, the efficacy and safety of CSA in combination with second generation H_1-antihistamines has been shown in both adult and pediatric populations.[6,7] CSA is considered as the fourth-line treatment after omalizumab in CSU since it is not licensed for urticaria and has an inferior profile of adverse effects.[8] According to the recent international EAACI/GA²LEN/EuroGuiDerm/APAAACI guideline, CSA is recommended only for patients with severe disease refractory to any dose of antihistamine and omalizumab in combination.[8] It is suggested to be used as the fourth-line therapy if the symptoms are intolerable or inadequately controlled within 6 months or earlier of omalizumab and high-dose antihistamines combination treatment.[8] CSA at low to moderate doses (up to 5 mg/kg body weight) are shown to be effective[6,7] and can directly decrease the release of mast cell mediators.[8] Its therapeutic effect is seen within 4–8 weeks.[9] The duration of CSA treatment in CSU is not well determined due to limited data. Depending on the patients' needs, it can be continued from 3 months to 3 years.[10] A meta-analysis and systematic review which included 18 studies with 909 CSU adult and pediatric patients from eight countries assessed the effect and safety of different doses and durations of CSA treatment.[7] They calculated the estimated response rate as 54.2%, 65.9%, and 73.1% at the 4th, 8th, and 12th weeks of the treatment respectively, indicating that the treatment of the patients whose symptoms do not resolve at the 4th week should be continued up to 12 weeks.[7] They also showed that CSA is effective at 2–5 mg/kg/day doses. According to the findings of this meta-analysis, adverse events are considered to be dose dependent regardless of the duration of the treatment and 3 mg/kg/day is shown to be a reasonable starting dose for most patients.[7] Although CSA seems to be an effective agent in CSU, it cannot be preferred to omalizumab due to its adverse effects such as renal toxicity, hypertension, hyperlipidemia, and gastrointestinal symptoms such as abdominal pain, nausea and vomiting, and neurotoxicity as well as the risk of malignancy.[4,7] The majority of these adverse events are mild and generally are reversible resolving after cessation or decreasing the dose.[7] Moreover, in a retrospective analysis, complete resolution was reported to be higher in patients who were treated with omalizumab than in those treated with CSA.[11] CSA should not be used in patients with any kind of malignancy, hypertension, and renal insufficiency.[12] However, the risk/benefit ratio of CSA is better than the long-term use of steroids.[8]

 ONLINE REFERENCES

To access the references of this chapter online, kindly refer to **emedicine360.com** also please follow the instructions mentioned on inside cover.

CHAPTER 14

Omalizumab

*Nasser Mohammad Porras,
Luis Felipe Ensina, Ana Maria Giménez-Arnau*

BACKGROUND

Chronic spontaneous urticaria (CSU) is a common disease with a prevalence of around 1%. It is characterized by wheals, angioedema, or both, showing a negative impact on quality of life. The international European Academy of Allergology and Clinical Immunology/Global Allergy and Asthma European Network/European Dermatology Forum/World Allergy Organization (EAACI/GA2LEN/EDF/WAO) urticaria guideline recommends a standard-dosed second-generation H_1-antihistamine as the first-line therapy.[1] However, this strategy is effective in <50% of patients. Up-dosing second-generation H_1-antihistamines up to four-fold can improve CSU response, although almost 40% of cases do not get adequate control of the disease. Omalizumab, a monoclonal anti-immunoglobulin E (IgE) antibody, was approved in Europe and the United States in 2014 for symptomatic moderate-to-severe CSU patients despite H_1-antihistamine treatment.[1,2] Clinical trials and real-life data have shown a good safety profile and efficacy in CSU treatment.[2-16]

MECHANISM OF ACTION

Omalizumab has been shown to improve symptoms of CSU, but its mechanism of action is not currently fully understood. Potential mechanisms include:
- Lowering IgE levels and downregulation of high-affinity IgE receptor (FcεR1).[17-19] These effects are observed earlier in basophils than in mast cells.[17,18]
- Reducing mast cell mediators' release. A reduction in the IgE bound to FcεR1 increases the mast cell degranulation threshold.[18]
- Reversing basopenia due to the recruitment of basophils to skin and improving basophil IgE receptor function, which is altered, provoking pathogenic histamine release.[18-21]
- Reducing activity of IgG autoantibodies against FcεR1 and IgE. Around 45% of patients with CSU/chronic idiopathic urticaria (CIU) have IgG autoantibodies against the α subunit of FcεR1, leading to activation of mast cells and basophils.[18]
- Reducing activity of IgE autoantibodies against an unknown autoantigen.[18] Up to 54% of patients with CSU/CIU have IgE autoantibodies against thyroid peroxidase (TPO).[18,22]

- Reducing activity of intrinsically abnormal IgE.[18] It has been described that abnormal IgE might contribute to symptoms in a subset of cold urticaria patients.[18,23]
- Decreasing the role of coagulation involvement. Tissue factors can induce the activation of eosinophils.[18]

CLINICAL DEVELOPMENT—CHRONIC SPONTANEOUS URTICARIA CLINICAL TRIALS

Efficacy

A systematic review for the EAACI Biological Guidelines evaluating the efficacy and safety of treatment with omalizumab for CSU was published in 2020. Nine randomized controlled trials (RCTs) (XTEND-CIU, POLARIS, Jörg 2008, GLACIAL, XCUISITE, ASTERIA I, MoA, MYSTIQUE, ASTERIA II, and X-ACT) performed between 2004 and 2017, including 1,620 patients with refractory CSU receiving omalizumab in addition to standard care versus placebo were selected. The range of treatment duration was between 4 and 24 weeks. The follow-up without medication ranged from 16 to 40 weeks. Only six studies included patients younger than 18 years old.[2]

Six studies showed that omalizumab at 300 mg every 4 weeks led to a clinically significant decrease in Urticaria Activity Score in 7 days (UAS7).[2,3] The same result was not observed with omalizumab at 150 mg every 4 weeks.[2,4] Eight RCTs evaluated the number of complete responders. For omalizumab 150 mg and 300 mg, an increased probability of achieving complete response compared to standard care was observed.[2]

Itching was evaluated by four RCTs with omalizumab 150 mg[2,5-8] and eight RCTs for omalizumab 300 mg[2-10,17] using Week Itch Severity Score (ISS7). In contrast to omalizumab 150 mg, omalizumab 300 mg was associated with a clinically significant reduction with a moderate evidence grade. In two studies, for both doses, a reduction in ISS7 was seen in patients 17 years old or younger.[2,8,10]

Dermatology life quality index (DLQI) was used to evaluate the quality of life in three RCTs with omalizumab 150 mg at week 12 and omalizumab 300 mg at week 24. DLQI was reduced only with omalizumab 300 mg, supporting that it may positively impact the quality of life, the reason why this is the licensed dose in Europe. One RCT showed a DLQI worsening of three or more points in the placebo group than in the omalizumab 300 mg group.[2] Other scores, such as Chronic Urticaria Quality of Life Questionnaire (CU-Q2oL), Work Impairment Score (WIS), and Activity Impairment Score (AIS), showed a significant improvement with omalizumab 300 mg.[2]

Five RCTs showed a diminished rescue medicine requirement at week 12 in omalizumab 150 mg and omalizumab 300 mg.[2]

Safety

Both doses might increase the risk of drug-related adverse effects (headache, asthenia, myalgia, injection-site reactions, and nasopharyngitis) with a low grade of evidence, as seen in three RCTs for omalizumab 150 mg and four RCTs for omalizumab 300 mg. However, omalizumab 300 mg might decrease with a moderate grade of evidence drug-related serious adverse effects. One study reported a case of anaphylactic shock.[2]

REAL-LIFE DATA–CHRONIC URTICARIA

Omalizumab for Chronic Spontaneous Urticaria in Real Life

Many studies confirm the usefulness of omalizumab in real life when treating CSU. We are reporting here some of them:

For instance, a systematic review and meta-analysis of 13 studies showed high-quality evidence that omalizumab effectively treats CSU in those patients refractory to antihistamine treatment compared to a placebo. The tools used to assess the effectiveness in the studies were UAS7, urticaria control test (UCT), and DLQI or CU-QoL. The best-observed dose was 300 mg. The adverse effect profile and a frequency similar to that observed in the placebo group confirm omalizumab safety in the recommended dosing regimen for CSU treatment. The primary adverse events were mild and included gastrointestinal manifestations, headache, the reaction at the application site, and skin changes.[24]

A Brazilian study evaluated 47 CSU patients treated with Omalizumab. Around 26 of 47 patients received Omalizumab at an initial dose of 300 mg/month. An improvement in urticarial symptoms was reported in the majority of patients. The 84.6% showed complete remission, and 4% partial remission. In eight patients with complete remission, the dose was reduced to 150 mg after 6 months, and the 50% of them had their symptoms controlled with this dose. Of the 20 patients who started Omalizumab 150 mg, the 60% had complete response. In six of the partial responders, a higher dose of 300 mg was used. Four patients had complete remission, two still had symptoms and the other two didn't have access to a higher dose. One patient did not respond to any dose. In conclusion, just one patient was considered as a nonresponder to Omalizumab, showing that it is a good treatment for refractory CSU.[25]

A study from Aarhus University Hospital with a total of 15 patients evidenced this. It included patients treated with omalizumab 150 mg every 4 weeks and 300 mg every 4 weeks. In case of no response, the dose was doubled, or the administration interval was reduced to 2 weeks. A significant decreased in the DLQI was observed during the first 2 months; later, it was stabilized. A significant reduction in UAS7 was seen as well. The UAS7 tended to increase in the last weeks of the injection cycle. None of the patients could stop H_1-antihistamine treatment. Paradoxically, IgE levels increased in some cases.[11]

Another study from Toronto University with 16 patients receiving omalizumab 150 mg every 2–4 weeks observed significant clinical improvement in 88% of cases. Ten cases experimented complete remission after the first injection (UAS7 = 0), two cases after the third injection, and two cases after the fifth and sixth doses. When evaluating long-term efficacy, only 3 out of the 14 patients who initially responded remained in complete remission without requiring maintenance treatment. In contrast, seven patients needed maintenance omalizumab, and one was in remission for 9 months since the last injection. Regarding systemic corticosteroid use, half of the patients could stop treatment with prednisone after starting omalizumab. Regarding adverse events, a brief flare of urticaria was observed in one patient at the first dose.[12]

A real-life survey from the Istanbul Faculty of Medicine with 14 patients receiving regimens as described before showed that omalizumab is also effective in treating angioedema manifestations. For instance, one patient never had more angioedema attacks since the start of omalizumab. As observed in the previous study, 12 patients responded almost after the first dose. In 14 patients, UAS7 and CU-Q2oL improved, persisting the response at 6-month control. Moreover, most cases reported no necessity of using H_1-antihistamine treatment. No adverse effects were observed.[13]

Finally, another retrospective study from Salman et al. with 106 patients with CSU showed a complete response (UAS7 = 0) in 50% of the patients and a well-controlled activity (UAS7 = 1 to <6) in 33% of the patients. An increased proportion of patients with a UCT ≥ 12 was observed. Moreover, higher rates of response were observed with omalizumab monotherapy compared to combination with antihistamines, and the combination with dapsone, colchicine, and omalizumab provided a benefit in a few numbers of patients.[14]

Omalizumab for Chronic Inducible Urticaria in Real Life

Omalizumab could have an essential role in the treatment of chronic inducible urticaria (CIndU) refractory to standard therapy. Many cases responding successfully to omalizumab have been published.

Metz et al. published a series of seven cases, including solar urticaria, cold urticaria, heat urticaria, delayed urticaria, and urticaria facticia confirmed by positive provocation test. All cases, before receiving omalizumab, previously received from 7 to 10 types of second-generation H_1-antihistamines as well as other treatments alone or in combination with H_1-antihistamines such as montelukast or antibiotics. In all cases, due to the refractory symptoms, omalizumab was started with different regimens. Only in two cases, the standard regimen of 300 mg every 4 weeks was initiated. Two cases were initially treated with 150 mg every 4 weeks; in one of these cases, the dose was increased to 300 mg every 4 weeks. Just one case was treated with 150 mg every 4 weeks. 5 of 7 cases responded, suggesting that omalizumab is also a good choice for treating CIU, although evidence is supported by case reports.[15]

A Catalan and Balearic Urticaria Network study with 80 participants with solar urticaria, cold urticaria, symptomatic dermographism, cholinergic urticaria, delayed pressure urticaria, aquagenic urticaria, and heat urticaria evaluated the therapeutic benefit of omalizumab for the different subtypes. In 75% of patients, a complete (UCT = 16) and satisfactory response (UCT ≥12–16) was observed. There were 22 nonresponders. Increasing the dose to 450 mg every 4 weeks led to a significant response in 14 of 22 nonresponders. With 600 mg every 4 weeks, four of the remaining seven nonresponders achieved satisfactory and complete responses. The response of patients with symptomatic dermographism was significantly more insufficient than those with solar urticaria or cholinergic urticaria. In 6 of 12 patients where omalizumab was stopped due to good disease control, omalizumab had to be reinitiated due to a relapse, again achieving a good response. In 57% of complete and satisfactory responders, the response was fast, with the fastest response rate for cold and solar urticaria.[16]

Other studies, including isolated case reports, have been published with the same results for treatment of cold urticaria, solar urticaria, delayed pressure urticaria, refractory severe heat urticaria, and cholinergic urticaria.[25-31]

HOW TO USE OMALIZUMAB IN CLINICAL PRACTICE

Indications in Dermatology
Treatment of CSU (and CIndU based on real-life data) refractory to a four-fold dose of H_1-antihistamine treatment.[1-2]

Initial Dosing
- Omalizumab 300 mg is administered subcutaneously every 4 weeks as an add-on therapy to high-doses second-generation H_1-antihistamines.[2]
- As a response to omalizumab is observed, H_1-antihistamines can be tapered down until the minimal effective dose.[2] Some patients will need no H_1-antihistamines to keep symptoms controlled after initiating omalizumab.[32]
- As anaphylaxis episodes have been reported with anti-IgE therapy but are rare. The safety profile observed in real-life use allows its use at home in some countries, when epinephrine autoinjector is available, after at least three doses administered in a hospital facility.[2]

Evaluation of Response
- After 4–6 months of initiating omalizumab, a response evaluation should be done.[33-35]
- The evaluation of response should be done combining disease activity data using UAS-7 (ideal objective: UAS-7 = 0), disease control data using UCT (ideal objective: UCT = 16), and a measure of quality of life, for example with DLQI. Until now, there are no validated criteria to define response to omalizumab.[33-35]
- It is essential to evaluate UAS7 weekly during all the month to have a global idea of whether the patient is adequately controlled or not.[33-35]
- Some predictors of response have been studied:[35]

	Fast response	Slow response	
Baseline total IgE levels[35-37]	High levels	Low levels	Type I autoimmunity
FcεRI high expression in blood basophil[38,39]	High levels	Low levels	
IgE anti TPO and IL-24[40]	High levels	Low levels	
IgG autoantibodies anti-TPO and anti-thyroglobulin[41]	Low levels	High levels	Type IIB autoimmunity
Positive basophil activation test[42]	–	+	
Positive autologous serum skin test[43]	–	+	
D-dimer[35]	Not useful	Not useful	

- Before starting treatment with omalizumab, such biomarkers could be considered to predict how CSU patients will respond to omalizumab.

Dose Adjustment–Clinical Scenarios

Based on the evidence of RCT and real-life data, the following approach could be adopted based on UAS7 score or UCT:[35,44,45]

- *Complete responder (UAS-7 ≤ 6)*: Two strategies can be done. Omalizumab dose could be diminished to 150 mg every 4 weeks and then stop if the patient is controlled with omalizumab 150 mg every 8 weeks. Another option is to prolong the administration interval to 6, 8, and 10 weeks and then stop. From real-life data, prolonging the interval of administration seems more beneficial.[28]
- *Partial responder (UAS7 7–16)*: Omalizumab 300 mg every 4 weeks must be maintained.
- *No responder (UAS7 >16)*: In this situation, an up-dosing strategy could be done based on clinical practice studies. The omalizumab dose can be increased to 150 mg every 3 months. The maximum dose that can be reached is 300 mg every 2 weeks or 600 mg every 4 weeks. If no response is seen with this dose, it is recommended to stop the treatment. The up-dosing strategy is especially successful in patients with body mass index (BMI) ≥ 30, an age >57 years, and those with previous treatment with cyclosporine.

Omalizumab is useful any time even a relapse of the CSU appears. A study showed that high baseline UAS7 and low UAS7 AAC (slow decrease of symptoms) indicate a higher probability of rapid symptom return than low baseline UAS7 and high UAS7 AAC.[46] Another study reflected that when relapsed, step-up to 300 mg helps a more significant proportion of patients achieve symptom control, and retreatment with omalizumab is as effective as initial therapy.[47]

Monitoring Laboratory Tests

No routine laboratory monitoring tests are recommended.

Adverse Events

- The most reported adverse events are headache, asthenia, myalgia, injection-site reactions, and nasopharyngitis.[48]
- Paradoxically, in <0.1% of patients, anaphylaxis has been described.[49] For this reason, it is recommended to administer the first three doses in a place with the necessary equipment and personnel to attend anaphylaxis with an observation period of 30 minutes. With proper patient education, the following doses can be administered at home, although it has not been licensed for home administration in all countries. As most cases of anaphylaxis are mild/moderate, discontinuation of omalizumab is not encouraged. On the other hand, professionals should report episodes of anaphylaxis for postmarketing surveillance.[48]

Combining Omalizumab with other Biological Treatments

A retrospective study reported the tolerability and safety of combining omalizumab with other biological therapies.[50]
- It included patients with age > 18 years receiving omalizumab combined with another biological treatment [anti-tumor necrosis factor (TNF) agents and secukinumab] for psoriasis, Crohn's disease, ulcerative colitis, and ankylosing spondylitis.[50]

- It showed that combined treatment was tolerated well. Moreover, no adverse events were detected, and no patient had to attend a hospital.[50]

Omalizumab, Infections, and Vaccines
- It is not recommended to stop it in case of active infection.[51]
- If the patient comes from an endemic area with a high incidence of geohelminths, pretreatment screening should be performed.[51]
- Vaccines should be administered 7 days before or after administration of omalizumab to address if adverse events are due to the vaccine or omalizumab.[51]

CONCLUSION

Omalizumab has been demonstrated to be the most effective treatment for moderate/severe CSU refractory to H_1-antihistamines. Its use is highly recommended once the correct diagnosis is made. Nevertheless, omalizumab does not completely control the disease in a percentage of patients, and its use can be required even for a long time. There is a place for further new treatments to be best than omalizumab is a challenge.

 ONLINE REFERENCES

To access the references of this chapter online, kindly refer to **emedicine360.com** also please follow the instructions mentioned on inside cover.

CHAPTER 15

Other Therapeutic Options

*Jesper Grønlund Holm, Paulo Ricardo Criado,
Roberta FJ Criado, Simon Francis Thomsen*

INTRODUCTION

In this chapter, we present other therapeutic options for patients with chronic urticaria (CU) in cases where guideline recommended therapies are unavailable, too expensive, have shown insufficient effect or have unacceptable side-effects.

RECOMMENDED TREATMENT OF CHRONIC URTICARIA

Treatment of CU follows the international guideline set by EAACI/GA²LEN/EuroGuiDerm/APAAACI.[1] First line of treatment is standard dose of oral, nonsedating, second generation antihistamines (sgH₁AHs). If symptoms persist, it is recommended to increase the dose of sgH₁AHs up to four-fold.[2] If symptoms still persist after 2–4 weeks, or are intolerable, add-on treatment with omalizumab [anti-immunoglobulin E (anti-IgE)][3] at a dose of 300 mg every 4 weeks is recommended. In refractory cases, dose of omalizumab can be increased up to 600 mg every 2 weeks but if symptoms remain despite this, it is recommended to discontinue omalizumab and use cyclosporine at doses up to 5 mg/kg body weight as add-on therapy to sgH₁AHs.

OTHER TREATMENT OPTIONS FOR CHRONIC URTICARIA

Various other nonbiologic, nonantihistamine therapeutic options exist, although the level of evidence for their efficacy and safety not met criteria for including them in the guideline recommendation. In the following we present an outline of treatments, which may serve as an alternative for guideline recommended treatments, sorted based on their usage and denoted with evidence levels when such are available (**Table 1**).[1]

Widely Used Treatments

Montelukast inhibits the leukotriene-D4-receptor, indirectly working as an anti-inflammatory drug, which is widely used in asthma, and still holds a place in the treatment of CU. Interestingly, apart from the existing evidence on the usage of montelukast for CU, several other studies have focused on paradox reactions to montelukast triggering urticaria symptoms.[10] All data considered, montelukast is a safe and extensively described treatment for CU, and serves as an alternative to

TABLE 1: Other therapeutic options for chronic urticaria.

Drug	Usage	Evidence for efficacy in CU
Anticoagulants (warfarin)	Infrequently	None
Anti-TNF-alpha inhibitors (etanercept, infliximab and adalimumab)[4]	Rarely	Very low
Autologous blood injection	Infrequently	Low
Azathioprine	Unrated	None
Colchicine	Rarely	None
Corticosteroids (systemic)	Unrated	None
Chloroquine/Hydroxychloroquine	Infrequently	Very low
Dapsone	Widely	Very low
Doxepin	Widely	Low
Dupilumab[5]	Rarely	Low
Heparin sodium[6]	Infrequently	Very low
Intravenous or subcutaneous immunoglobulin (IVIG)	Infrequently	None
Immunomodulating drugs	Rarely	Low
Methotrexate	Widely	Very low
Mepolizumab[7]	Rarely	None
Montelukast	Widely	Moderate
Mycophenolate mofetil	Widely	None
Plasmapheresis	Infrequently	None
Pseudoallergen-free diet	Widely	Low
Ranitidine/Cimetidine[8]	Widely	None
Ruxolitinib (Janus Kinase inhibitor)[9]	Very rarely	None
Sulfasalazine	Widely	None
Tacrolimus	Very rarely	None
Tranexamic acid	Infrequently	None
PUVA	Infrequently	Low
UVB	Infrequently	Low

(CU: chronic urticaria; TNF: tumor necrosis factor; UV: ultraviolet light; PUVA: psoralen + UVA)

Source: Modified from Zuberbier T, Aberer W, Asero R, Abdul Latiff AH, Baker D, Ballmer-Weber B, et al. The EAACI/GA2LEN/EDF/WAO guideline for the definition, classification, diagnosis and management of urticaria. Allergy 2018;73:1393-414.

biologic therapy, when this is not available, although it is markedly less effective.[11] The overall evidence level for its use is considered moderate.

Dapsone is a sulfone antibiotic drug, mainly targeting neutrophil inflammation, which has been extensively used for a range of dermatoses, including lepra, pemphigus vulgaris, pyoderma gangrenosum,[12] dermatitis herpetiformis, and acne.[13,14] Less than ten studies have described the use of dapsone for CU, however, with the majority of patients reporting good to complete effect of the treatment. Few side-effects from treatment are reported, including hypersensitivity and livedo reticularis,[15,16] however, the risk of hemolysis should always be considered. In a nonblinded prospective trial, 22 CU patients were allocated for distinct drug use according to their histopathological findings on urticaria biopsies; 4 patients received a regimen of antihistamines plus dapsone 100 mg/day (predominantly neutrophilic dermal inflammatory infiltrate) during 2 months, and the authors observed complete resolution of hives and itch. Other 9 patients received colchicine, due to some contraindication for dapsone use (8 patients demonstrated complete resolution of their CU).[17] A small randomized controlled trial (RCT)[18] compared dapsone + desloratadine to desloratadine alone and found no additional effect from addition of dapsone to desloratadine. Therefore, dapsone appears safe and somewhat effective, although antihistamines alone match the potential effect, leaving the overall level of evidence very low for dapsone therapy.

Methotrexate is a folic acid antagonist with anti-inflammatory, antiproliferative, and immunomodulatory properties. However, the mechanism of action in CU is not entirely known, and the limited evidence for its use is based on case studies and a small RCT, which found no significant effect on urticaria symptoms compared to placebo. Therefore, the overall level of evidence is very low, and considering the potential liver toxic effects from methotrexate and the continuous monitoring required, it is fit as a treatment for CU is circumstantial.[19,20]

Doxepin is a tricyclic antidepressant with antipruritic properties, mainly used for major depression and anxiety. Although few RCTs have been conducted on its use for cold urticaria, showing moderate efficacy, the overall level of evidence for its use is considered low.

Pseudoallergen-free diet is widely used to treat or control symptoms in numerous conditions, including CU. However, low level of evidence supports its use, and it can therefore, not be considered an evidence-based treatment modality.

Ranitidine and *cimetidine* are H_2-antihistamines, which are often used for insufficiently controlled CU. However, robust trials testing H_2-antihistamines as add-on treatment in patients unresponsive to H_1-antihistamines are warranted.

Mycophenolate mofetil is an immunosuppressive drug, which inhibits deoxyribonucleic acid (DNA) synthesis in lymphocytes. Originally, used to prevent rejection in organ transplant recipients, mycophenolate mofetil has also been used for treatment of atopic dermatitis and psoriasis. Little data exists on its use in CU, limited to a few case series,[21-24] however, all reporting positive to complete effects from treatment without any side-effects. However, the limited number of reported cases and the lack of larger randomized trials, question the wide use of mycophenolate mofetil for CU.

Sulfasalazine is an antibacterial sulfa-drug belonging to the DMARD (disease-modifying antirheumatic drugs) group of drugs. Originally developed for the treatment of rheumatoid arthritis, sulfasalazine has since been explored as an immunosuppressant, used in combination with azathioprine in organ transplant recipients. Numerous noncontrolled studies have investigated the use of sulfasalazine in CU with mainly positive effects. Notably, several reports of severe side-effects, including leukopenia and rhabdomyolysis were reported,[25,26] advocating a limitation of its use.

Infrequently Used

Ultraviolet (UV) light can act as trigger of urticaria symptoms in patients suffering from solar urticaria. Reactions can be in response to UVA (380–320 nm), UVB

(320–280 nm), visible light (700–390) or a combination of these.[27-29] In patients with other forms of CU, theoretically, irradiation of the skin with UV-light can elevate the threshold for elicitation of symptoms, thus increasing patients' ability to expose their skin and minimizing symptoms. Published data from an RCT on the use of UVA or UVB in patients with CU has found that a large proportion of the patients experienced milder pruritus and whealing, as well as improved quality of life after treatment with either psoralen + UVA or UVB.[30] However, the overall evidence level for the use of UVB compared to psoralen + UVA (PUVA) is low, whereas, compared to sgH$_1$AHs it is considered very low. In addition, UV treatment has not been shown to be a valid long-term treatment option in CU.

Chloroquine and *Hydroxychloroquine* hereof act as histamine antagonists and are mainly used for malaria and rheumatic diseases. The mechanism of action of chloroquine makes it a relatively safe alternative with potential efficacy in CU.[31,32] However, few studies have been published, limiting the evidence of its use. Notably, a small RCT found improvement in quality of life, but no significant clinical improvement in specific urticaria scores.[33] Therefore, the level of evidence for chloroquine remains very low.

Anticoagulants, mainly the vitamin-K antagonist, warfarin, and used for thrombosis prophylaxis, have been reported as a treatment option for CU. However, no larger trials exist leaving little evidence to support its use.

Tranexamic acid is used against hemorrhage in surgical specialties acting as an antifibrinolytic drug. Documentation for its effect in hereditary angioedema has pointed to its potential for CU and angioedema. Flares of CU/angioedema have been shown to be followed by increased thrombin generation, fibrinolysis, and inflammation, supporting possible benefit from tranexamic acid use.[34,35] One double-blinded study found no superior effect from tranexamic acid compared to placebo,[36] however other, smaller, nonblinded reports have found a beneficial effect from treatment, although indicating no effect from repetitive usage.[35,37-39] Seemingly, the potential effects of tranexamic acid are inefficiently documented to merit recommendation.

Intravenous immunoglobulin G (IVIG) is an antibody product obtained from healthy donors. The mode of action is not entirely understood but is believed to be a combination of inhibitory effects on B-cell and/or T-cell functions. The use of IVIG in CU has been extensively described, however without any RCTs published. The effect of IVIG appears to be good, with numerous cases of complete remission of symptoms reported, despite frequent side-effects.[40,41] In addition, IVIG relies on advanced technological equipment and set-up, making it highly expensive and unavailable in most centers.

Plasmapheresis is based on filtration and clearance of plasma, and is widely used for treatment of autoimmune diseases, and could potentially be beneficial in CU. However, few smaller case reports exist, which fail to show consistent and reproducible effect from plasmapheresis. Also, plasmapheresis is expensive and requires specialized equipment, limiting its use to very few centers. Based hereon, despite its theoretical potential, plasmapheresis hardly has a place in the treatment of CU.[42]

Autologous blood injection has been compared to placebo in a small number of RCTs in patients with CU, although without results to support a desirable effect, leaving a low certainty of evidence for its use.

Rarely Used

Immunomodulating drugs, including cyclophosphamide, rituximab, anakinra, anti-TNF, and camostat mesilate, are all used to treat autoimmune diseases. Although CU is increasingly considered a disease of autoimmune origin, no controlled trials on the potential benefit of these treatments in CU exist, leaving low level of evidence to support their use.

Colchicine is an alkaloid drug, with anti-inflammatory properties used in the treatment of gout. A handful of uncontrolled studies have been published on its use in CU, showing overall good effect, with the majority of patients showing remission of symptoms. However, gastrointestinal symptoms are a prevalent side-effect of colchicine.[43]

Very Rarely Used

Tacrolimus acts as a calcineurin inhibitor, thus sharing properties with cyclosporine, and is used to prevent organ rejection in transplant recipients. However, its use in CU is not supported by any trials.

Unrated

Azathioprine is a cytostatic drug widely used for immunosuppressive purposes. Uses include atopic dermatitis and urticarial vasculitis, and in organ transplant recipients. A few controlled and uncontrolled studies have shown good effect from azathioprine use in patients with CU, however, no large RCTs exist. Based on the available data azathioprine appears safe and could serve as an alternative for insufficiently controlled CU. However, its definite recommendation awaits further trials.[1]

Corticosteroids are successfully used in many allergic diseases. In CU, a short-course of systemic corticosteroids is recommended in cases of sudden flares to control otherwise intractable symptoms.[44] It is very important to avoid long-term use of systemic corticosteroids due to the metabolic side-effects and challenges with withdrawal. There is no evidence to support use of topical corticosteroids in CU.[1]

CONCLUSION

New and effective treatments for CU, particularly omalizumab, have been introduced in the past decades with newer targeted treatments underway. However, various factors, primarily national reimbursement regulations and economy, can limit the availability and use of guideline recommended treatments. Numerous potential alternatives exist, although with little evidence for their efficacy and safety. However, the existing data suggests safe and efficient alternatives, which could be used in recalcitrant cases, where omalizumab treatment has failed or is unavailable. Such use should be extensively monitored with protocolled publication of data to strengthen our knowledge on those other therapeutic options less well described.

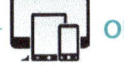 ONLINE REFERENCES

To access the references of this chapter online, kindly refer to **emedicine360.com** also please follow the instructions mentioned on inside cover.

CHAPTER 16

Treatment Algorithm for Chronic Urticaria

*Ismahaan Abdisalaam, Tessa Niemeyer-van der Kolk,
Désirée Larenas-Linnemann, Martijn van Doorn*

STEPWISE TREATMENT OF CHRONIC URTICARIA

Patients with chronic urticaria are treated using a stepwise approach according to the severity and course of the disease (**Flowchart 1**).[1] Ultimately, the goal of the treatment is complete symptom relief and disease control. As first step (1a), patients are treated with a second generation H_1 antihistamine in the registered dose (usually once daily). It should be noted that first generation antihistamines (e.g., hydroxyzine and clemastine) have anticholinergic and sedative properties and should therefore, be avoided in the treatment of chronic urticaria (for details also see chapter on treatment with antihistamines). In case of insufficient response or intolerability, a change to another second generation H_1-antihistamine can be considered. If the prescribed antihistamine does not provide adequate symptom relief after 2–4 weeks, or earlier in case of very high disease activity, the next

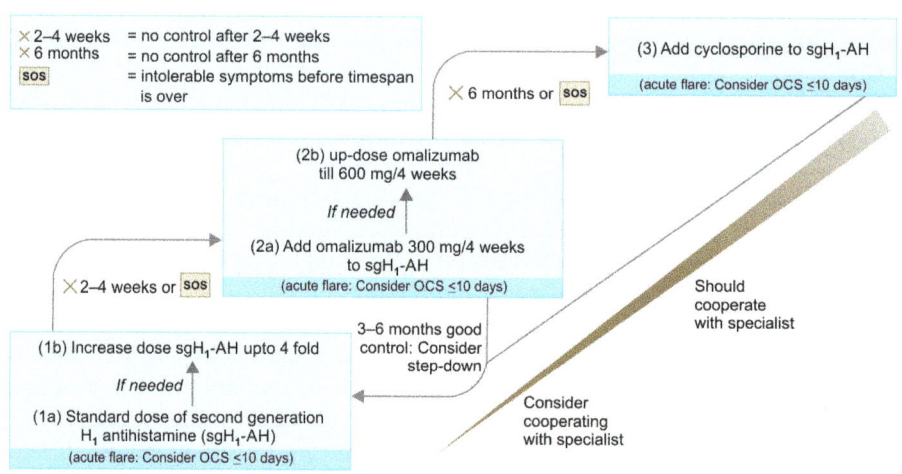

(SOS: As required; OCS: Oral corticosteroids; SgH1 AH: Second generation H1 antihistamine)

FLOWCHART 1: Stepwise approach for the treatment of chronic urticaria.

Source: Adjusted from reference 1.

treatment step can be taken. As studies have shown a clear benefit of up-dosing second generation H_1-antihistamines up to four-fold in patients not responding to the registered doses this is treatment step 1b.

Prescribing antihistamines in doses up to four-fold of the standard dose is off label and thus patients need to be well informed about the potential side-effects. For most patients, there is sufficient data indicating that long-term continuous use of H_1-antihistamines is safe and from real world experience it is known that higher doses are generally well tolerated by the patients.[2,3] Caution is advised up-dosing elderly patients, since some sedative effects can still occur, even with second generation antihistamines. Patients experiencing sedation or drowsiness after up dosing can be treated with the second generation antihistamines that exhibit less sedation: Fexofenadine and bilastine.[4,5] Relative contraindications for up dosing of antihistamines include patients with known long QT-syndrome, or concomitant use of drugs that prolong the QT-interval as this may result in cardiac arrhythmias (also see chapter treatment with antihistamines).

The add-on therapy of a leukotriene receptor antagonists (e.g., montelukast) has been omitted from the stepwise approach in the international guidelines due to the limited evidence for its clinical benefit.[1] However, due to the high costs and limited availability of omalizumab (step 2) in some countries, it could still be considered as treatment option since it can be (partially) effective in individual patients.

Nonresponders to treatment step 1b should be referred to a specialist (dermatologist or allergist) for treatment with omalizumab. Omalizumab is a humanized anti-immunoglobulin E (IgE) monoclonal antibody, which is safe and effective in chronic spontaneous urticaria (CSU) and is also reported to be effective in several types of chronic inducible urticaria (CIndU).[6-8] The recommended starting dose is 300 mg subcutaneous every 4 weeks, although the licensed dose and maximum treatment duration can vary between countries. For example, in some countries the recommended starting dose is 150 mg and dose escalation up to 300 mg can only be performed in unresponsive patients. Analogous to the second generation H_1-antihistamines omalizumab can be given safely as long-term treatment and can eventually be up-dosed to 600 mg every 4 weeks (step 2b), see also 'Dose escalation'. Omalizumab is also effective and safe in patients with histaminergic angioedema and has shown to drastically improve patients' quality of life.[9]

If treatment with omalizumab is not effective or cannot be tolerated, cyclosporine should be considered as the next step treatment option (step 3). Cyclosporine is effective and has a direct effect on mast cell mediator release, but is known for its high incidence of adverse effects (e.g., gastrointestinal upset, hypertension, and renal toxicity). Its use in patients with chronic urticaria is off label, and is therefore only recommended for patients with severe disease not responding to any dose of H_1-antihistamines and omalizumab. However, long-term treatment with cyclosporine is still preferred over the continuous use of oral corticosteroids because of their well-known serious long-term side effects. However, for acute urticaria and exacerbations of CSU a short course of corticosteroids (i.e., 20–50 mg/day for 5–10 days) can be used safely.[1]

DOSE ESCALATION AND PERSONALIZED OMALIZUMAB TREATMENT

In the registration studies for omalizumab dose maintenance, up- or down-dosing, and treatment discontinuation have not been investigated. In the international guidelines dose optimization for omalizumab has been formally discussed and an up-dosing recommendation is given if standard dosing is not sufficiently effective after months. However, according to the label, for urticaria omalizumab has a fixed dosing schedule and hence treatment cannot be tailored to the needs of the individual patient, which is a major limitation. Therefore, several real-world studies have investigated the effects of off label up-dosing as well as down-dosing in patient with chronic urticaria.[10,11]

An example of a recently published treatment algorithm which includes up- and down-dosing of omalizumab is shown in **Flowchart 2**. According to this algorithm,

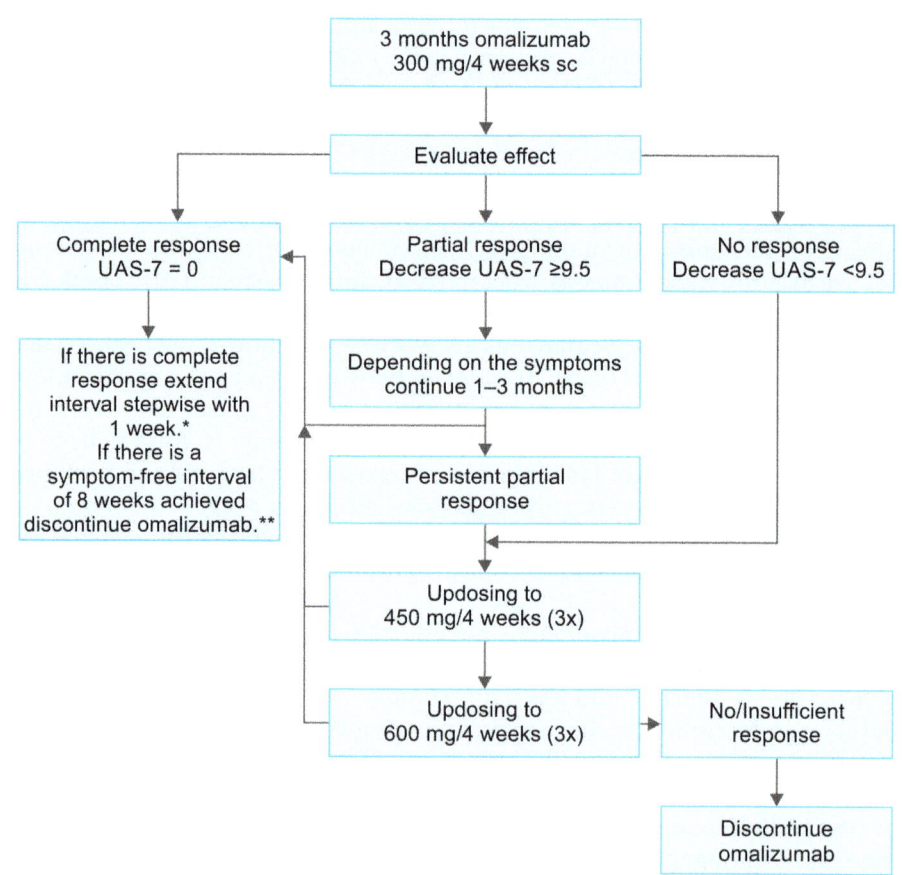

Note:
* Before extending the interval for partial responders who are symptom-free on a higher dose, stepwise down-dose to a standard dose of 300 mg/4 weeks.
** Restart omalizumab if relapse occurs after discontinuing the treatment.

(UAS7: 7-day urticaria activity score activity score)

FLOWCHART 2: Personalized omalizumab treatment algorithm.

omalizumab should be up-dosed or the dosing interval shortened (e.g., 3 weeks and 2 weeks) in patients who do not achieve complete remission with the standard treatment regimen (300 mg/4 weeks). Also, to balance the cost-effectiveness of this approach, omalizumab should be down-dosed (i.e., gradual prolongation of the dosing interval) and eventually discontinued in patients who have achieved a durable complete remission. The effectiveness of this algorithm in a clinical setting was evaluated by Niemeyer–van der Kolk et al. and the reported efficacy rates in this study (77.8% complete responders and 17% partial responders) were considerably higher than the response rates with omalizumab per label at 300 mg/4 weeks as well as the response rates in clinical trials.[12] Also, the long-term complete remission rates after tapering (58% achieved long-term remission) were greater than reported in previous omalizumab stop-studies.[13,14] A personalized treatment approach may lead to better individual outcomes and should therefore be considered in clinical practice.

OMALIZUMAB TREATMENT IN PATIENTS WITH CHRONIC INDUCIBLE URTICARIA

At present, omalizumab is only licensed for the treatment of asthma and CSU. However, there is a growing body of evidence supporting the use of off label omalizumab in CIndU patients in whom the disease has a large impact on their quality of life and in whom the CIndU is refractory to treatment with (escalated doses of) H_1-antihistamines.[15] In addition, there is new real-world evidence that up-dosing omalizumab in patients with CIndU who have a suboptimal response at 300 mg/4 weeks can be beneficial.[16]

CONCLUSION

In summary, according to the international guidelines, patients with chronic urticaria are treated using a stepwise approach. After initiation therapy with a second-generation antihistamine (step 1a), the next step is up-dosing to a four-fold dose (step 1b). Preferably this dose escalation is performed by their treating family physician. If a patient remains symptomatic after up-dosing of antihistamines, referral to a specialist for treatment with omalizumab (second step) is indicated. Finally, up-dosing of omalizumab or shortening of the dosing interval can be considered in patients who are not or partially responding to the standard dose or dosing interval.

 ONLINE REFERENCES

To access the references of this chapter online, kindly refer to **emedicine360.com** also please follow the instructions mentioned on inside cover.

CHAPTER 17

Urticaria in Children

*Connor Prosty, Sofianne Gabrielli, Michelle Le,
Elena Netchiporouk, Moshe Ben-Shoshan*

INTRODUCTION

Consistent with the definition in adults, pediatric urticaria is defined by the presence of pruritic wheals and/or angioedema. Urticaria is classified based on duration of symptoms into acute urticaria (AU) (<6 weeks) and chronic urticaria (CU) (≥6 weeks). Among pediatric patients, AU is more prevalent than CU.[1] Pediatric CU, like adult CU, is subclassified into chronic inducible urticaria (CIndU) and chronic spontaneous urticaria (CSU), based on the ability to identify a specific trigger. Pediatric CU presents as urticaria alone in 78.4%, angioedema alone in 6.6%, and urticaria and angioedema in the remaining 15% of patients (**Fig. 1**).[2]

Current studies and guidelines on urticaria predominantly focus on adults. We aim to identify noteworthy differences and knowledge gaps existing between pediatric and adult urticaria.

PREVALENCE AND NATURAL HISTORY

A meta-analysis determined that the point prevalence of CU among children is 1.43% compared to 0.86% in adults.[3] As opposed to adult CU that is more common

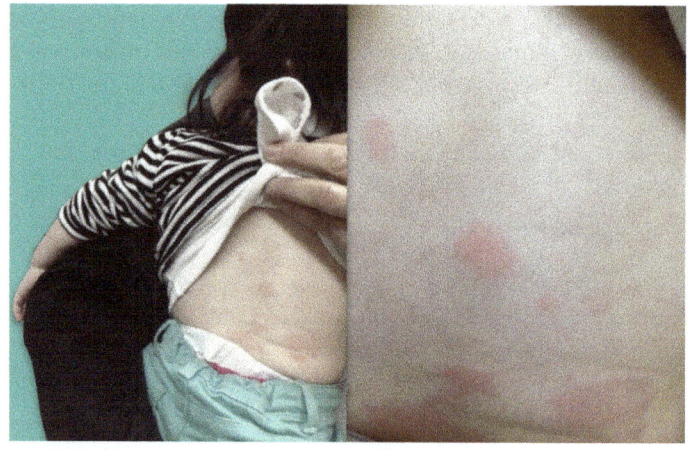

FIG. 1: Chronic spontaneous urticaria (CSU) presenting with wheals in an infant.

among females, the prevalence is similar in males and females in children <15 years old.[3] The median age of onset of pediatric CU is 5–9 years.

The resolution of pediatric CU (defined as 1 year without wheals in the absence of treatment) is 10.3%/year.[4] Specifically, in children 45.3% of CIndU cases resolve in 6 years[5] and 50% of CSU cases resolve in 5 years.[6]

Acute Urticaria

Pediatric AU is reported in up to 13.9% of children and often leads to emergency room visits.[1] Etiologies of AU in children presenting to the emergency room include: infection (51.26%; respiratory, gastrointestinal, unidentified, and otitis media), idiopathic (34.37%), inhaled allergens (6.99%), drugs (4.08%), food (2.52%), and insect stings (0.78%).[7] The majority of AU cases can be managed by non-sedating antihistamines and only a minority progress to CU.[8]

Chronic Spontaneous Urticaria

Chronic spontaneous urticaria accounts for the majority of pediatric CU cases.[4] Overall, the pathogenesis of pediatric CSU is thought to be similar to adult CSU, albeit it remains understudied. In approximately half of children, an autoimmune etiology is suggested, whereas the remaining cases are thought to be idiopathic.[9] In line with the autoimmune hypothesis, autoimmune diseases (i.e., hypothyroidism, lupus, juvenile arthritis, and type 1 diabetes mellitus) are more common among pediatric CSU patients than the general population of pediatric age, which is consistent with adult CSU.[10]

Chronic Inducible Urticaria

Chronic inducible urticaria is less common than CSU and accounts for approximately 20% of pediatric CU cases.[4] Up to a third of pediatric CIndU patients have concomitant CSU.[4] Similar to adults, pediatric CIndU is diagnosed by provocation test and is classified into physical and nonphysical forms.[11]

Physical Chronic Inducible Urticaria

Symptomatic dermographism (SD) is characterized by the development of pruritic wheals at sites of skin friction or rubbing (**Fig. 2**). SD accounts for approximately half of pediatric CIndU and 40% of cases are reported to resolve within 5 years.[12]

Cold urticaria is the development of wheals and/or angioedema in response to cold objects, air or water (**Fig. 3**). Cold urticaria prevalence is highly variable, accounting for as much as 71% of pediatric CIndU.[4] Cold urticaria has a poor prognosis in both adults and children, with resolution rates in children reported as low as 20% in 5 years.[12] Anaphylaxis has been reported in approximately a fifth of pediatric cold urticaria cases and epinephrine autoinjector prescription may be considered.[8] Importantly, cold urticaria starting in childhood needs a thorough history taking to rule out mimicking genodermatoses such as *PLCG2*-associated antibody deficiency and immune dysregulation, and cryoprin-associated periodic syndromes.[8]

Solar urticaria is triggered by light exposure (ultraviolet and/or visible) and accounts for up to 6% of pediatric CIndU.[5] In children, it is associated with a poorer resolution rate than other types of CIndU.[5] Notably, erythropoietic protoporphyria,

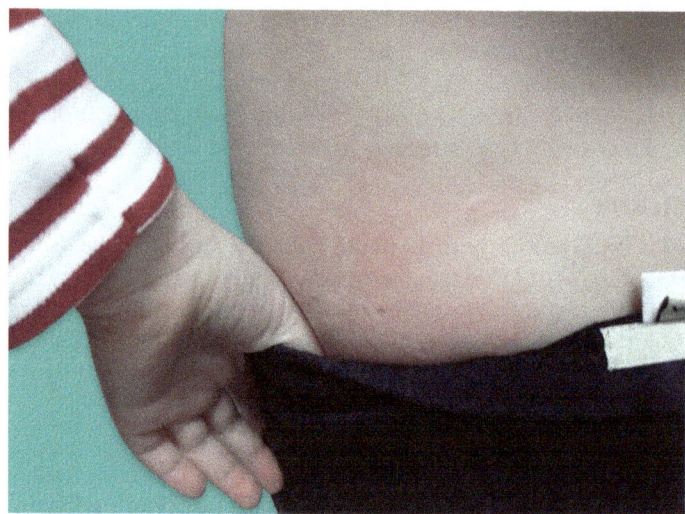

FIG. 2: Symptomatic dermographism (SD) in an adolescent.

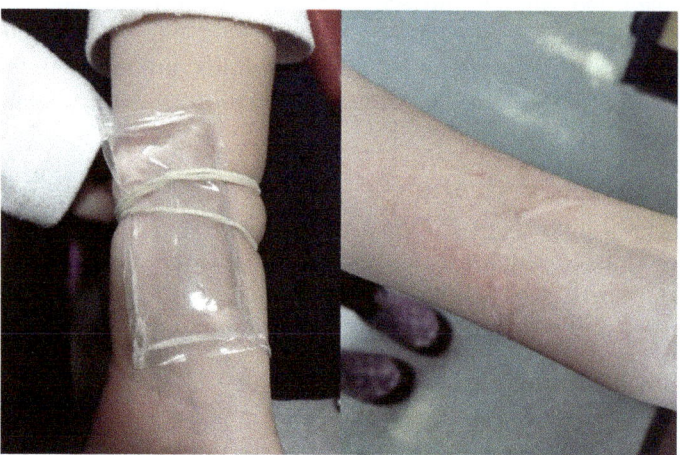

FIG. 3: Ice cube test performed on an adolescent patient with cold urticaria (left) and wheal response to cold provocation test (right).

hydroa vacciniforme, polymorphous light eruption, and actinic prurigo are similarly appearing photodermatoses that should be included in the differential diagnosis.[12]

Vibratory, heat, and delayed pressure urticaria are triggered by vibration, heat exposure, and sustained pressure to the skin, respectively. They are extremely rare and scarce data is available on their prevalence and prognosis in children.[12]

Nonphysical Chronic Inducible Urticaria

Cholinergic urticaria is the development of small pruritic wheals from an increased core body temperature through exercise or passive warming. The prevalence of cholinergic urticaria among pediatric CIndU ranges up to 42%.[5] It has a poor prognosis in children, with one study reporting only 1/11 (9%) patients symptom-free after 4.5 years of follow-up.[12]

Contact and aquagenic urticaria are triggered by contact with an offending agent and contact with water, respectively. Data on pediatric contact and aquagenic urticaria are sparse due to their rarity.[12]

ASSESSMENT TOOLS

Currently, there are no validated severity scores or disease control scores for children diagnosed with CU. The Urticaria Activity Score (UAS) is the guideline-recommended gold-standard for disease activity for adults with CSU.[13] Several case reports and pediatric cohort studies have proposed the potential use of weekly UAS (UAS7) in children, while other authors have adapted the scoring of the UAS7 for reduced body surface area in children.[13] In two large pediatric studies, elevated UAS7 at baseline was associated with persistence of urticaria symptoms[14] and with the need for treatment with omalizumab.[15] However, larger-scale studies are required to validate the use of UAS7 in children. The Urticaria Control Test (UCT) was validated for use in patients 12 years and older, demonstrating a high degree of reliability and validity and strong correlation with UAS.[16]

In patients presenting predominantly with recurrent angioedema with or without the presence of wheals, the Angioedema Activity Score (AAS) and the Angioedema Control Test (AECT) should be used for disease assessment.[17] Similar to the UAS7 and UCT, these tools remain to be validated in the pediatric population.

The Children's Dermatology Life Quality Index (CDLQI) has been validated for use in CU for ages 4 years and older;[18] however, a limitation of these tools is the lack of disease-specific questions. As such, the Chronic Urticaria Quality of Life Questionnaire (CU-Q2oL) was developed to assess quality of life impairment, specifically in CU patients and has been validated for use in adults.[19] As studies on children are currently lacking, the CDLQI remains the best tool for quality of life assessment among children with CU.

Management

Antihistamines

Treatment algorithms for children with CU have largely been extrapolated from adult guidelines. Current European Academy of Allergology and Clinical Immunology (EAACI) guidelines recommend a stepwise approach in which second-generation H_1-antihistamines are the first-line treatment in children.[11] Numerous studies have established the efficacy and safety of second-generation H_1-antihistamines in children older than 2 years, which include cetirizine, desloratadine, fexofenadine, levocetirizine, rupatadine, bilastine (approved in Europe for children 6 years and older), and loratadine.[8,9,13] Randomized-controlled trials (RCTs) comparing the effectiveness of various antihistamines versus placebo in children determined that in all cases, the groups treated with antihistamines were statistically superior in improvement of symptoms and quality of life compared to placebo groups[8]. First-generation H_1-antihistamines for the treatment of CU in children are discouraged as they are poorly selective against H_1 receptors and can easily cross the blood-brain barrier, increasing the likelihood of adverse events, including cognitive impairment.[9]

If symptoms of CU are not adequately controlled within 2-4 weeks, second-line treatment involves up-dosing second-generation H_1-antihistamines up to four-fold the licensed dose.[11] The efficacy of dose escalations has not been properly established in children and is recommended on the basis of studies conducted in children with rhinitis.[8] However, RCTs conducted in adolescents and adults using four-fold dose of second-generation H_1-antihistamines demonstrated efficacy and safety.[8]

Omalizumab

Guidelines recommend omalizumab as third-line treatment for CSU in adults. While the majority of pediatric CU cases are controlled with second-generation H_1-antihistamines,[15] omalizumab is approved for use in children 12 years and older with CSU or combined CSU and CIndU.[13] Among adolescents and adults, omalizumab is well-studied. Use of omalizumab is reported to reduce UAS7 with good tolerability.[8] Off-label use in patients <12 years of age has been reported in several case reports and in a subset of patients among cohort studies.[8] Due to small samples size and lack of any RCTs in children, the level of evidence is low, although the majority of studies report improvement in symptoms.[15] Elevated UAS7 at baseline and presence of cholinergic urticaria were predictors of requiring treatment with omalizumab in pediatric CSU.[15] Omalizumab is also considered off-label treatment in cases of CIndU; however, prior reports in adults and children suggest safety and efficacy in those with severe CIndU, which typically do not respond well to antihistamine treatment.[5]

Other Treatments

Cyclosporine in addition to antihistamines is recommended if omalizumab fails to control CU. Guidelines recommend cyclosporine as last option as its use is limited by its possible side-effects,[13] which include risk of decreased renal function and hypertension in a dose-dependent manner.[15] Careful monitoring of cyclosporine serum concentration among patients is required during treatment.[9] Few studies have assessed treatment with cyclosporine in children aged 9 years and older. The majority of children reported control of symptoms without significant adverse events.[9] However, the level of evidence for cyclosporine use in children remains low.

The use of steroids in children with CU should be discouraged except for short-term use (up to a maximum of 10 days) to treat severe exacerbations.[13,15] There is risk of significant side effects in children, such as behavioral abnormalities, adrenal suppression, and avascular necrosis, with long-term management with corticosteroids.[8,15]

Other monoclonal antibodies are currently emerging as potential therapies for pediatric CSU. A recent RCT using ligelizumab excluded children; however, there are four active clinical trials which include adolescent patients.[9] Dupilumab was used as treatment in two children presented in a case series by Staubach et al. The patients had failed therapy with omalizumab followed by cyclosporine; one patient showed significant improvement with dupilumab treatment after 1 month and the other patient, after 3 months.[20]

CONCLUSION

In summary, CU is not a rare entity in children and has no sex predilection. While CSU is more common than CIndU, identifying whether a trigger exists is the first step to manage and prevent CU. Studies are required to establish the pathogenic mechanisms of CU in children and to assess the risk of other autoimmune diseases. Current management is limited to avoidance of identified triggers in CIndU cases, treatment with second-generation H_1-antihistamines and, for pediatric patients over the age of 12 years, omalizumab in poorly controlled cases. Future studies investigating the safety and efficacy of omalizumab and other biologics for patients with CSU under 12 years and validating the use of assessment tools will contribute to better management of pediatric CU.

 ONLINE REFERENCES

To access the references of this chapter online, kindly refer to **emedicine360.com** also please follow the instructions mentioned on inside cover.

CHAPTER 18

What is New in Urticaria? Pathophysiology

M Sendhil Kumaran, Vignesh Narayan

PATHOGENESIS OF URTICARIA

INTRODUCTION

Urticaria is a common disease, with a prevalence of 0.7% across all age groups. It is almost equally as prevalent among children as it is among adults. Although there is a higher prevalence among women in the adult age group (1.3% vs. 0.8%), it is the reverse in children with boys being more affected than girls (1.1% vs. 1%).[1] Available studies show that there is an increasing trend in the number of cases of uricaria point prevalence with the passage of time.[2,3] Thus, there is a need to better understand its pathogenesis, so that we may be better equipped to predict its behavior and brandish new modalities of therapy. The following **Flowchart 1** elucidates the pathogenesis in a brief manner:

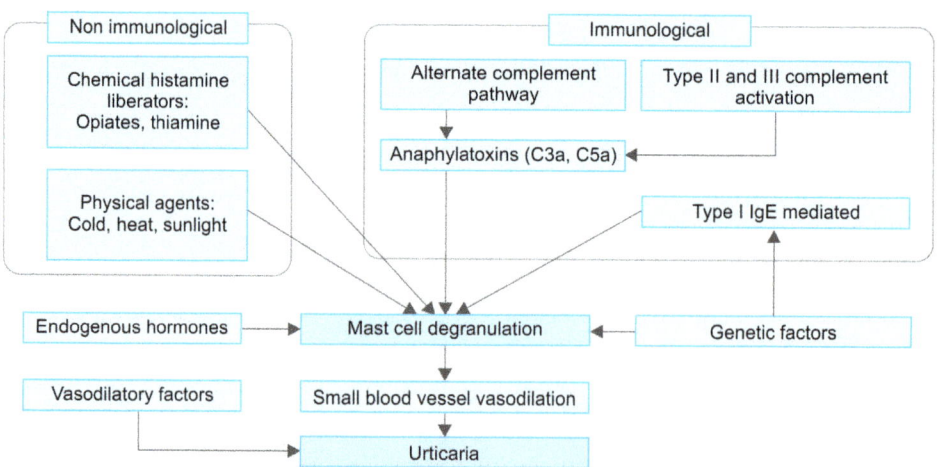

FLOWCHART 1: Showing pathogenesis of urticaria.

MAST CELLS

Mast cells are white blood cells found in throughout the body, being most avidly present in the skin, blood vessels, lungs, and intestines. They possess high affinity IgE receptors (FcεRI) on their surface and degranulate, releasing a plethora of mediators on stimulation bringing about the whole cascade of urticaria. They are the main culprits implicated in the pathogenesis of urticaria. There are two types of mast cells: Those which possess tryptase and chymase and those with tryptase alone. The latter are found in bowel, alveolar, and the nasal mucosa; whereas more important to us is the former-being localized in skin and intestinal mucosa. Mast cells are however, thought to be involved in innate immune response, wound healing, and neuroendocrine function, and are thus not vestigial.[4]

Mast Cell Degranulation

The cascade of events leading to degranulation of mast cells can begin either with IgE receptor mediated or independent mechanisms. The former may be initiated by the cross linking of receptor bound IgE by an allergen, or via the presence of anti-FcεRI antibodies. This snowballs into calcium and energy dependent steps causing release of mediators. However, not all individuals with these antibodies have urticaria and these antibodies have been found in individuals without urticaria, such as those with lupus erythematosus. This led to search for other nonantibody-mediated mediators of release. Few of these molecules are such as opiates, substance P and anaphylatoxins, and stem cell factor.[5]

The following **Figure 1** elucidates the various mechanisms for mast cell degranulation:

Mediators Released

Upon stimulation, there is a bombardment of preformed mediator release, along with the slow synthesis and release of newly formed mediators. The major share of the pre-formed mediator is histamine, with smaller contributions from proteases, heparin, and histamine. Also released are cytokines such as tumor necrosis factor (TNF), granulocyte-macrophage colony-stimulating factor (GM-CSF), and

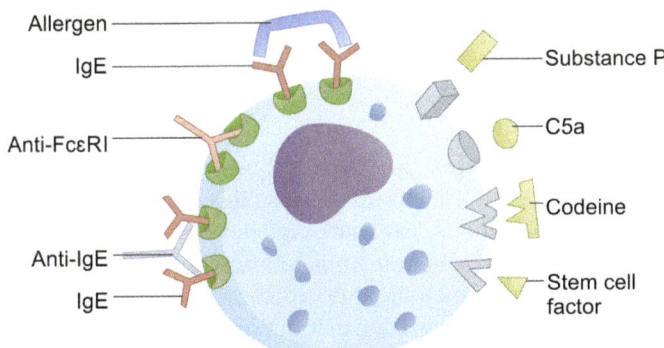

Stimuli for degranulation of mast cells

(FcεRI: fragment crystallizable epsilon receptor 1; IgE: immunoglobulin E)

FIG. 1: Stimulating factors of mast cells.

interleukins 3, 5, 6, 8, and 13. Newly formed mediators include eicosanoids such as prostaglandin D_2 and slow reacting substance of anaphylaxis (constituted by leukotriene C_4, D_4, E_4).[6]

Blood Vessels

The fusillade of inflammatory mediators dilates blood vessels, principally the postcapillary venules leading to plasma leak. Simultaneously there is upregulation of adhesion molecules and chemotactic signals into the wheal of urticaria.[7]

Blood

Autoantibodies

The FcεRI receptor has an α1 subunit and an α2 subunit. The former allows for the binding of autoantibodies in a noncompetitive manner, even in the presence of IgE, whereas IgE competes with the binding of the latter. A third mechanism that circumvents the receptor binding is antibodies against IgE itself. These in turn push the dominos of complement activation in motion via the C5a anaphylatoxin, which fuels the ongoing fire. There have also been described nonIgE mediated mast cell liberators. These antibodies may serve as a useful marker as they correlate with disease severity.[8]

Leukocytes

Basophils are thought to keep the engine running in urticaria, by releasing mediators like histamine. These basophils however are unique in that they have been found to have reduced response to anti-IgE. This is thought to be due to increased negative regulatory protein SHIP (src homology 2-containing inositol phosphatase). This has especially been seen in the active phase of the disease, with the response to anti-IgE improving, with clinical recovery. In contrast to the peripheral blood picture, eosinophils are increased in wheals. They possibly keep the torch burning via secretion of slow reacting substance of anaphylaxis.[9]

Nerves

The increased secretion of substance P and other neuropeptides have proven to show a wheal and flare response upon intradermal injection, similar findings have also been found in vitro. Patients with urticaria also had a greater wheal response compared to those without, upon injection of vasoactive intestinal peptide.[10]

Mechanism of Urticaria

Exogenous allergens cross link the already bound IgE to FcεRI, and is more implicated in the acute than the chronic forms. This is probably best represented from urticaria to latex, and foods. The role of IgE has been studied in cold and solar urticaria, although the exact mechanism is unknown. Implicated are neoantigen formation and presentation. In cholinergic urticaria, there may be factors released by nerve endings or a sweat allergy. Gain of function mutation in adhesion G protein E_2 has been implicated in pressure induced and vibratory urticaria.

In case of spontaneous urticaria, it is due to leakage of plasma. In fact, increased plasma levels of D-dimer and prothrombin fragments have been demonstrated.

Food additives and nonsteroidal anti-inflammatory drugs divert prostaglandins into leukotrienes.

Mast Cell Independent Urticaria

These do not involve mast cells, ergo their management is different. Nonimmunological contact urticaria to benzoic acid is suppressed with nonsteroidal anti-inflammatory medications. In autoinflammatory syndromes with urticaria, there is improvement with the administration of interleukin-1 receptor antagonists. Bradykinin levels are elevated and are implicated in the pathogenesis of angiotensin-converting enzyme (ACE) inhibitor induced urticaria.[11]

Types of Urticaria

Urticaria is mainly of two types: Type I and type IIb, based on the underlying mechanism.

In type I urticaria, there is the presence of IgE antibodies against an allergen, which after binding leads to degranulation. Further research has divulged the antigenic autoallergenic target to be thyroid peroxidase, thyroglobulin, tissue factor, double stranded deoxyribonucleic acid (dsDNA), and interleukin-24. Studies have shown that incubation of the basophils from patients with this type of urticaria with thyroid peroxidase and interleukin 24 ex vivo, led to massive degranulation. The therapeutic implication of this being that targeting these antibodies, with agents such as omalizumab and ligelizumab may cure these patients. These patients, in fact, have been shown to have a better response and chance to cure compared to the other subtype. These patients also have a higher rate of concomitant allergies.[12]

Type IIb subset of urticaria patients have IgG, IgM, and IgA against the FcεRI present on basophils and also against IgE. Most pathogenic being IgM, higher levels being linked to higher disease activity, lower basophil and eosinophil count. The serum of these patients is capable of activating heterologous basophils to degranulate. These patients are also autologous serum skin test (ASST) positive. These patients tend to be refractory to therapy with anti-IgE antibodies and have a protracted course of illness.[13,14]

Receptors and Signaling Molecules

Our recent understanding of the tug of war between stimulatory and inhibitory molecules in the signaling pathway of mast cells have led to the discovery of newer therapeutic options.

Extracellulary: Alarmins, thymic stromal lymphopoietin innate immunity enhancing cytokines (IL25, IL33) are elevated in urticaria. Mast cells depend on KIT for survival, and could be a potential target. Complement receptor blockade could also shut down the machinery.

Intracellularly: The downstream signaling can be blocked by targeting Bruton tyrosine kinase. Coinhibitory receptors like Siglec 8 and CD 200Ra targeting is also an option.[15]

DIAGNOSIS AND TREATMENT OF URTICARIA

Guillet Carole, Leu Noemi, Schmid-Grendelmeier Peter

DIAGNOSIS

In routine diagnostics of patients with chronic spontaneous urticaria (CSU), recent guidelines generally recommend limited tests (differential blood count, C-reactive protein, and/or erythrocyte sedimentation rate) and extended diagnostics only depending on the patient's history.[1] By asking the right questions at the initial encounter, patients in whom further investigations should be performed have to be identified. A recent consensus-based article compiled a series of questions that can be asked when taking a history of an urticaria patient in order to identify patients requiring additional diagnostic measures.[2] As per this expert panel recommendation, specialists should measure total immunoglobulin E (IgE) and IgG anti-thyroidperoxidase (TPO), and asses for type I and type IIb autoimmunity by using basophil activation testing.[2,3] Furthermore, these experts recommend D-dimers and total IgE to be tested in order to be able to better predict treatment response and disease duration.[2,4,5]

TREATMENT

The primary principle when treating chronic urticaria (CU) is to eliminate symptoms, including pruritus, wheals, and angioedema.[6] H_1-antihistamines function as inverse agonists of the H_1-receptor and are a well-established base of urticaria treatment. However, <50% of patients have complete control of symptoms with licensed doses of H_1-antihistamines[7] and four-fold antihistamine dosing is insufficient in 54% of patients with CSU.[8] In patients unresponsive or only partially responsive to standard and four-fold antihistamine dosages, according to European consensus guidelines, addition of omalizumab, an IgG-anti-IgE monoclonal antibody (mAb), is indicated and approved for those over 12 years since 2014. In patients refractory to high-dose antihistamines and omalizumab, standard immunosuppressive agents should be used according to guidelines (e.g., cyclosporine).[1,6] Various treatments (mAbs, small molecules and also topical agents), partially already licensed for use in other diseases, are under investigation for use in CU/CSU and shall be briefly discussed in this chapter.

Off-label use of Treatments Licensed for the Treatment of Other Diseases than Chronic Urticaria

Mepolizumab, Benralizumab, and Reslizumab

Eosinophils are thought to play a role in the pathogenesis of CU and are present in lesional and nonlesional skin of CSU patients.[9,10] Mepolizumab, reslizumab, and benralizumab, [anti-interleukin (IL-5) and anti-IL-5 receptor mAbs] were successfully used for the treatment of patients with CSU in case reports or case series.[11-13] The efficacy of benralizumab and mepolizumab is currently being evaluated in CSU trials (NCT03494881, NCT03183024).

Dupilumab

Many CSU patients have elevated IgE levels and sensitizations to autoallergens implying Th2-driven disease mechanisms. Consequently, targeting Th2-specific cytokines such as IL-4 and IL-13 has led to a reduction of CSU symptoms in some patients treated with the fully human mAb dupilumab directed against the IL-4 receptor alpha subunit.[14] There are several ongoing phase II and III randomized controlled trials (RCTs) (NCT03749135, NCT04180488) evaluating the use of dupilumab in CSU.

Secukinumab

In lesional and nonlesional skin of CSU patients, elevated IL-17A levels have been found and in a small case series of eight CSU patients improvement of symptoms upon treatment with the humanized mAb secukinumab directed against IL-17A was found.[15] Currently, there are no ongoing trials with anti-IL17A mAbs in CSU.

Rituximab

Rituximab is a chimeric mAB directed against CD-20 surface on B-cell receptors leading to B-cell depletion. The rationale for using rituximab in CSU is the presence of IgG against the high affinity IgE-receptor (FcεRI), therefore, rituximab may be of use in cases of type IIb autoimmune CSU.[16] To date, there are only case reports describing the beneficial effect of rituximab in CU.[17,18] Currently, no trials with rituximab in CSU are ongoing.

Antitumor Necrosis Factor Alpha

In skin biopsy specimen of urticaria patients, TNF-α can be elevated and thus, anti-TNF-α mAbs may present a treatment target.[19] Treatment success in delayed-pressure type CU and in difficult to treat CSU was reported in single cases and case series.[20,21]
Currently, no trials with anti-TNF-α mABs in CU are ongoing.

Novel Treatments under Development for use in Chronic Spontaneous Urticaria and Mast Cell Diseases

Ligelizumab (QGE031)

Ligelizumab is a humanized IgG1k antibody that binds IgE with high affinity. Ligelizumab binds an epitope that only partially overlaps with that of the marketed anti-IgE antibody omalizumab, which has lower affinity to the target IgE.[22] As a consequence of their molecular differences, the two antibodies have distinct inhibition profiles. In a phase 2-dose finding trial (n = 382), a higher percentage of patients treated with ligelizumab had complete control of symptoms of CSU with ligelizumab therapy of 72 mg or 240 mg than with omalizumab or placebo.[23] The safety and efficacy of ligelizumab in the treatment of CSU in adolescents and adults inadequately controlled with H_1-antihistamines is currently being evaluated in two randomized, double-blind, active- and placebo-controlled phase 3 studies (NCT03580369, NCT03580356). The estimated primary completion date of both studies is in mid-2021.[24]

AK002: A Humanized Monoclonal Antibody to Siglec-8

Siglecs (sialic acid binding immunoglobulin-like lectins) are surface proteins expressed on immune cells. Siglec-8 is selectively expressed on the surface of mast cells, eosinophils, and basophils.[25] By targeting Siglec-8, AK002, a humanized mAb, mast cell activity can be inhibited and eosinophils depleted.[26] A phase 2a, open-label pilot study of the safety and efficacy of AK002 in patients with CSU and cholinergic urticaria (NCT03436797) demonstrated activity in all forms of CU, including omalizumab-refractory cases and is now ongoing in an extension trial. It has shown potential for patients suffering from CU, including those refractory to antihistamines and omalizumab.[27]

Inhibitors of Type 2 Immunity-inducing Cytokines/Tezepelumab (AMG 157)

Thymic stromal lymphopoietin (TSLP), IL-33 and IL-25 are epithelial cell derived cytokines initiating type 2 immunity leading to production of IL-5, IL-9, and IL-13. These cytokines have effects on mast cells and are relevant in the pathogenesis of CSU.[9,28] Tezepelumab is a human mAb inhibiting the action of TSLP. It has been shown to be efficacious in the treatment of asthma and leads to a reduction in total serum IgE levels.[29] Tezepelumab is under investigations as a treatment for CSU in a phase 2b study (NCT04833855). IL-33, IL-25, and TSLP are potentially suitable candidates to be targeted by novel treatment strategies of CSU.

Bruton's Tyrosine Kinase-inhibitors (Remibrutinib (LOU064) and Fenebrutinib (GDC-0853))

Bruton's tyrosine kinase (BTK) plays a pivotal role in the signaling cascade downstream of the FcεRI and the B-cell receptor. BTK is essential for FcεRI-mediated mast cell activation and for the maturation and functioning of B cells. Treatment with a BTK inhibitor inhibits IgE- and mast cell dependent responses in mice and humans.[30] BTK-inhibitors are usually administered orally twice daily. Fenebrutinib and remibrutinib are being tested in clinical phase 2 trials for use in CSU (NCT03137069, NCT03693625, NCT03926611, and NCT04109313).

CRTh2 Antagonist (AZD1981)

Prostaglandin D_2 (PGD_2) is secreted by mast cells upon activation and leads to eosinophil and mast cell chemotaxis via its receptor chemo-attractant receptor-homologous molecule expressed on Th-2 cells. In CSU, expression of CRTh2 on basophils and eosinophils is reduced, potentially due to PGD_2 effects.[31] A phase 2 RCT evaluating the effects of the selective CRTh2 antagonist AZD1981 on symptoms in patients with H_1-antihistamine refractory CSU showed reduction of itch, PGD_2 induced eosinophil shape change, and increased eosinophil count.[32]

Topical Spleen Tyrosine Kinase Inhibitor (GSK2646264)

Spleen tyrosin kinase (Syk) is a tyrosine kinase in the FcεRI pathway promoting mast cell degranulation and histamine release. It has been implicated in CSU pathogenesis.[33-35] The small-molecule Syk inhibitor (GSK26462649) applied topically in a cream inhibited histamine release by human skin mast cells in situ.[35] A phase 1 study investigating the safety, local tolerability, pharmacokinetics, and pharmacodynamics after topical application of GSK2646264 in healthy individuals and with CSU was recently completed (NCT02424799). The results are expected to be published soon.

Future Directions in Chronic Urticaria Treatment, Diagnosis, and Pathogenesis

Chronic urticaria is a debilitating and often poorly controlled disease. Currently, antihistamines and omalizumab are the only licensed treatments. Additional and better treatments are required. Off-label treatments with mAbs targeting Th-2 cytokines (dupilumab) and IL-5/IL-5R (mepolizumab and benralizumab) are currently in RCTs for CU. Other IgE-targeted antibodies than omalizumab (ligelizumab) with higher affinity are in phase 3 trials. Other promising drugs including small molecules and topical agents are under development and partially

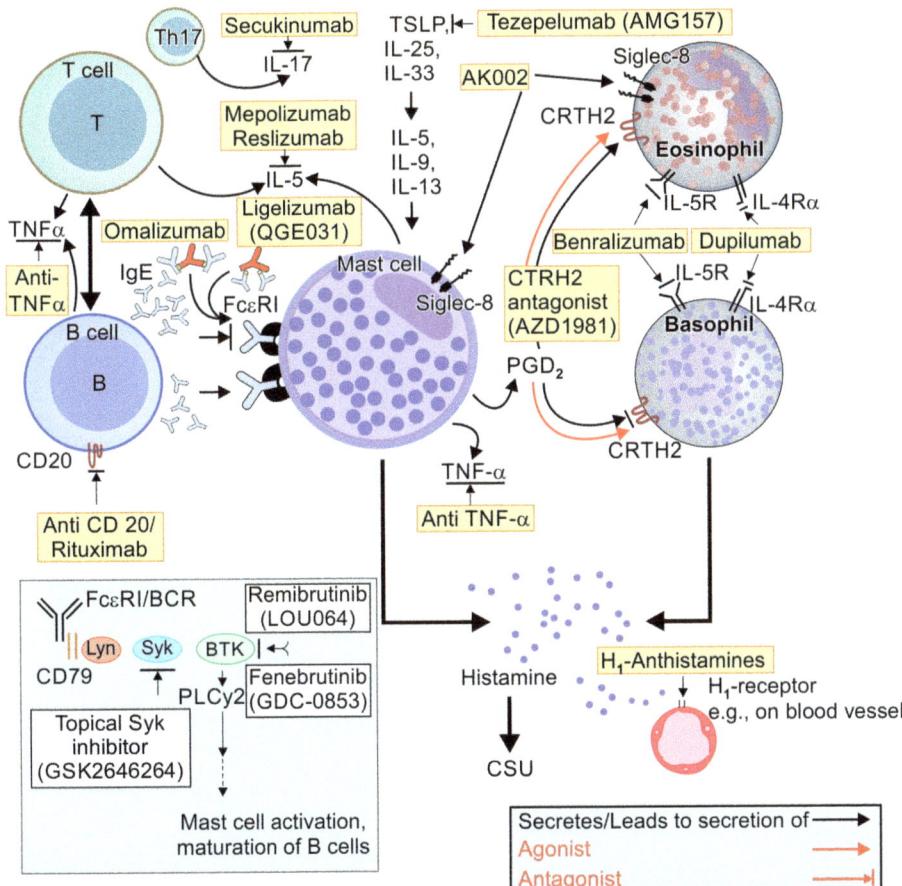

(CSU: chronic spontaneous urticaria; FcεRI: fragment crystallizable epsilon receptor 1; IL: interleukin; TNF-α: tumor necrosis factor-α)

FIG. 1: An overview of potential target molecules in the pathogenesis of chronic urticaria and future targeted therapies.

in clinical trials. To date, all current treatments for CU are aimed at controlling the disease and preventing its signs and symptoms, not curing it. Further studies should explore potentially curative treatment options and therefore better understanding of disease mechanisms are needed.

Potential target molecules in the pathogenesis of CU and future targeted therapies are shown in **Figure 1**.

 ONLINE REFERENCES

To access the references of this chapter online, kindly refer to **emedicine360.com** also please follow the instructions mentioned on inside cover.

CHAPTER 19

Patient Education Material

Hermenio Lima, Iman Hamed Nasr, Naoko Inomata

INTRODUCTION

Patient–doctor or patient-health system relationships are complex. Patients may feel intimidated in a formal healthcare setting and are not constantly communicating with their physician or healthcare provider about their behaviors. Furthermore, physicians have a limited amount of time to spend with patients. It is not always evident that the medical information provided is understood and will be placed into practice.[1] There are language and cultural differences that aid miscommunication.[2] Therefore, many physicians rely on patient education material (PEM) to fill this interaction gap and encourage patient engagement in the treatment prescribed, especially in chronic diseases.[3]

Chronic urticaria (CU), an exchangeable term for chronic spontaneous urticaria (CSU), is not the most common type of inflammatory skin disease. However, its prevalence varies between 0.1 and 1% during the lifetime in a different part of the world.[4] Nonetheless, the disease causes a significant impact on patients' social, economic, quality of life, and well-being. Despite efforts by health organizations, research centers, healthcare providers, and physicians to encourage early detection and treatment of CU, many never have treated this condition even in its most severe presentations. Part of this could be associated with the lack of excellent and effective PEM for CU.

Patient education materials have been approached to provide updated information with medical precision and scientific evidence toward the disease on focus. The PEMs format has always been positive in creating a better interaction with the population recipient, even to somewhat modify the health provider style of communications from the physician's point of view. Nonetheless, they fail to be remembered or to direct changes in subjects' behavior with the idea of improving treatment engagement. They cannot direct changes on subjects' adherence to behavioral changes.[5]

Medical literature about PEM for CU is scarce. Here, we discuss the rationale, the principles, and the premises on which a future material could be conceived in the field. Such an approach should recognize the emotional components of human behavior in the presence of chronic inflammatory disease and used appropriate advertising principles targeting patient engagement and persistence toward CU treatment.

WHAT ARE PATIENT EDUCATION MATERIALS?

Patient education materials function. Patient education allows patients to understand their disease better and to cope positively with urticaria. Patients with CU need long-term care, which can stretch from months to years. Therefore, patient self-management is as essential as the doctor's day-to-day guidance and treatment. PEMs can be quickly introduced in clinical settings. They will help to improve their knowledge of their disease and skills in self-management, even though patients feel anxious to ask questions or do not visit their doctors.

Principles for writing PEMs. Information in PEMs should be based on scientific evidence and should cite guidelines. Personal experience and opinions should be avoided as much as possible. However, if needed, it would be better to specify it as an opinion to avoid confusion. In addition, PEMs should be as straightforward as possible and should be written in plain language, avoiding medical terms.

Contents and means of providing PEMs. PEMs are provided by individual healthcare providers, such as doctors and nurses, public institutes, academic associations, pharmaceutical companies, and patient associations. The topics of PEMs are diverse, ranging from general information about urticaria to self-management and strategies for self-management to the various coping challenges patients face. PEMs also include information in the form of handouts from healthcare workers, DVDs, and online sites. In terms of content complexity, online materials are easily accessible to patients through sites such as YouTube. For example, allergy United Kingdom (UK), a leading national charity, provides support, advice, and information for those living with allergic disease, such as urticaria and educational materials online, including leaflets and YouTube videos in English. The British Association of Dermatologists (BAD) offers patient information leaflets.

The patient education materials assessment tool (PEMAT) and user guide were recently introduced.[6] PEMAT is a systematic method to evaluate and compare the understandability and actionability of patient educational materials. It is intended as a general guide to help determine whether patients can comprehend and take action on data. Separate instruments are available for use as printed and audiovisual materials.

PATIENT EDUCATION MATERIALS MODELS

What are Hives (Urticaria)?

Hives or medically known as urticaria, are raised areas of the very itchy, reddish or light-colored skin (**Figs. 1A** and **B**). These raised areas may enlarge and merge. Angioedema is swelling that happens in the face, eyelids, ears, mouth, hands, feet, or genitals with discomfort in the swelling area. The skin area is usually expected in color, but there may be slight redness of the skin in some cases (**Fig. 1C**). Angioedema may occur alone without the hives. Hives can occur with or without angioedema.

Hives develop when specific immune cells in the body called mast cells get activated, releasing chemicals such as histamine, causing itching, redness, and swelling. Hives appear suddenly and disappear within several hours (<24 hours). They may appear once again in other areas of the body.

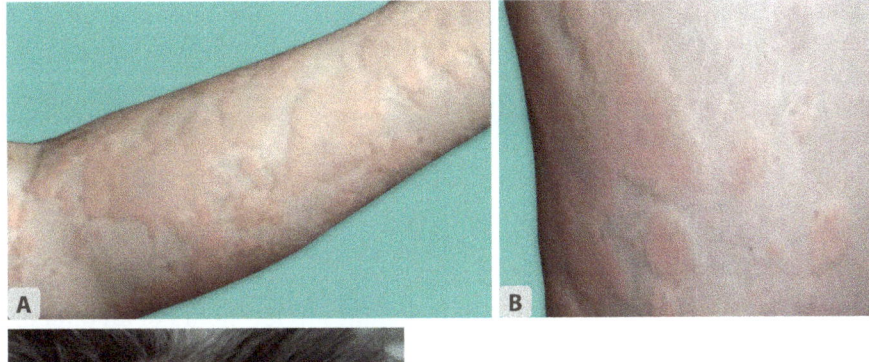
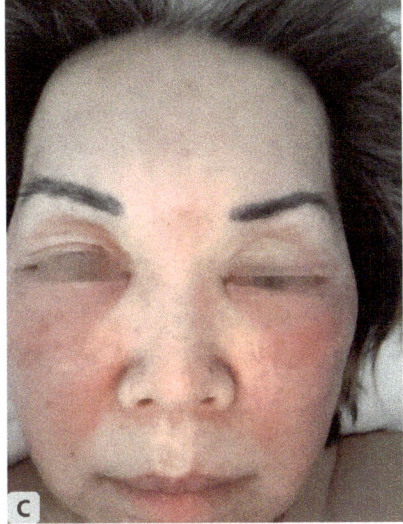

FIGS. 1A TO C: A patient suffering from urticaria (raised areas of the very itchy, reddish or light-colored skin).

Hives are a common condition. Around 1 in 5 people will have hives at some time during their lives. They may be mild (nonbothersome), moderate (bothersome but does not interfere with daily activities or sleep), and severe (bothersome interfering with daily activities or sleep)

Contact your doctor if you have severe pain, bruising of the skin, lesions lasting >24 hours, tiny purple or red colored spots, or fever that occur along with hives as these are not typical features of hives and might point to a different condition.

What are the Types and Causes of Urticaria?

It is essential to understand the types of urticaria or hives to determine their cause. These types are: (1) Acute urticaria—brief/sudden hives either once or on and off; (2) Chronic urticaria—long-term, on and off, lasting >6 weeks; (3) Inducible urticaria—triggered by certain types of physical stimulation, such as heat and pressure.

Acute hives (acute urticaria). Most hives are acute that occur suddenly and will not last beyond a few days (maximum 6 weeks). Triggers may be allergic or nonallergic. It is crucial first to exclude an allergic reaction as acute hives may be a part of a severe allergic reaction (anaphylaxis) that may be life-threatening, if untreated.

You should see a doctor as soon as possible if you develop hives or angioedema suddenly, alone or along with other symptoms, such as:
- Difficulty or trouble breathing.
- Wheezing or whistling sound in the chest.
- Tightness in the throat.
- Feeling lightheaded or dizzy.
- Nausea or vomiting.
- Cramping abdominal pain.
- Collapse, loss of consciousness.

These symptoms usually occur within minutes to few hours of an offending trigger, such as:
- *Drugs*—antibiotics, pain killers, anesthetics, and contrast dyes used in imaging.
- *Insect stings*—bees, wasps, and fire ants.
- *Food allergies*—common foods that cause allergy are: peanuts, nuts, shellfish, eggs, wheat, milk, soy, and fish. Typically appear within an hour of eating the food. It may occur as late as 4 hours as in red meat allergy.
- *Physical contact*—hives after touching certain substances you are allergic to (nuts, animals, plants, and latex).

Other triggers of acute hives (nonallergic) can include the following:
- *Infections*: Viral infections are the most common cause of acute urticaria in children. The hives appear around 1 week or more after the illness begins and disappear after 1-2 weeks.
- *Insect stings*: Hives around the area of the sting only.
- *Idiopathic (no trigger identified)*: This type of acute urticaria is called acute spontaneous urticaria and may occur once or on and off but usually not lasting beyond 6 weeks.

Chronic hives (chronic urticaria). CU tends to come and go on most days for 6 weeks or more, sometimes for years. They are very itchy and may occur with or without angioedema or as angioedema alone. They typically appear and disappear in less than a day and significantly interfere with sleep and daily activities such as work or school.

In most cases of CU, the cause is unknown and nonallergic. It can be a sign of other medical or autoimmune conditions such as thyroid disease, lupus or chronic infections. Most people with one of these conditions will have other symptoms apart from hives.

Chronic urticaria's common triggers include heat, cold, stress, alcohol, tight fitting clothes, an infection, lack of sleep, spicy food, and some drugs such as aspirin and ibuprofen.

If your hives get worse when you eat certain foods or take certain medications, try to avoid those and see if your symptoms go away. You need to consult your doctor. It is imperative to pay attention to your symptoms to exclude an allergic cause for your hives.

Chronic urticaria can be frustrating as it affects how an individual looks and is unpredictable, so they fear when the next attack will happen. In many cases, they avoid many foods unnecessarily, thinking they may be causes. People may avoid you because of the fear that it is contagious.

The good news is that allergies rarely cause CU, are not life-threatening, not contagious, and are treatable in most people. They are rarely permanent; almost 50% of people are hive-free within 1 year, others may last a few years. Learning what triggers your hives can help you avoid the trigger and avoid the hives.

Inducible hives (inducible urticaria). These are hives that form in response to various physical stimuli such as pressure, heat, or cold. They tend to be long lasting for years and are considered a type of CU.

The most common causes of inducible hives include:
- *Stroking*: Raised lines on the skin along with areas that have been stroked or scratched (skin writing or dermatographism).
- *Pressure*: Swelling anywhere on the body that has been pressed on (after few hours of applying the pressure), such as swelling of the palms when carrying a heavy object, swelling of the feet after walking long distances or wearing tight shoes.
- *Cold*: Hives that develop when cold skin warms again. This type may cause a severe reaction (anaphylaxis) if you go for swimming in frigid water.
- *Increased body temperature or sweating*: These are tiny and numerous and appear on reddened skin when they cool off after a hot shower or cool down after exercise.
- *Vibration*: Hives on parts of the body that have been touching something that vibrates (after holding onto the steering wheel while driving, mowing the lawn or using the jackhammer).
- *Exercise*: Hives when cooling down after exercise. However, if the hives show up during exercise, this can be a sign of a dangerous condition called exercise-induced anaphylaxis and requires immediate attention by your doctor. It is essential to stop and rest as soon as you develop hives. Continuing to exercise can be very dangerous.
- *Sunlight*: Hives following direct exposure of the skin to sunlight (rare)
- *Water*: Hives with direct skin contact with water (rare).

Do I need Tests for Hives?

The diagnosis is usually based on the symptoms and physical examination. For acute hives, allergy testing may be recommended if concerns about allergies as a cause of symptoms and referral to an allergist are vital. For chronic hives, blood tests are sometimes done to look for a possible association, such as thyroid disease. Other considerations.

Skin biopsy: Rarely, a sample of the affected skin is removed (skin biopsy) to help identify causes of nontypical hives (severe pain, bruising, concomitant fever, or those that last more than a day). It may also be done if blood tests are abnormal.

Tests for inducible hives: This is performed by recreating the conditions that cause the hives. They are helpful to diagnose the condition and also to monitor the response to treatment.

How are Hives Treated?

- *Avoidance of triggers*: This is the first and most critical step in the treatment of hives. If the trigger is known, you need to avoid it.

- *Medications*:
  - *Antihistamines*: These are medicines that can relieve itching and reduce swelling. Most people respond to antihistamines. You may need a higher dose to control your symptoms. They work better if you take them regularly. The newer antihistamines such as (cetirizine, loratadine, fexofenadine, desloratadine, and levocetirizine) are better for treating hives because of their longer duration of action and fewer side effects than older antihistamines (chlorpheniramine maleate, hydroxyzine, and diphenhydramine that may cause drowsiness and dry mouth).
  - *Oral steroids*: Steroids are sometimes given short-term if antihistamines alone do not relieve severe acute hives and are stopped once the hives have improved. Prolonged use of steroids for months or years can lead to side effects (high blood pressure, diabetes, and weight gain).
  - *Other treatments*: There are additional treatments such as omalizumab and cyclosporine if your hives do not get better with the antihistamines. Omalizumab is added to the antihistamines and is given by allergists and dermatologists as monthly injections.

What about Urticaria in Pregnancy and Breastfeeding?

Hives in pregnancy vary; they may flare, stay the same or get better. In some cases, it may worsen following delivery. You need to consult an allergist or dermatologist. If you experience flare-ups, certain treatments can be given during pregnancy and lactation without risk to the baby, such as some new antihistamines (loratadine, cetirizine, desloratadine, and levocetirizine). Old antihistamines should be avoided. Studies showed that omalizumab is safe in pregnancy as well as in breastfeeding if required.

INFORMATION TECHNOLOGY FOR PATIENT EDUCATION MATERIAL AND CHRONIC SPONTANEOUS URTICARIA

Information technology has transformed the decision-making process for clinicians and offers new possibilities for healthcare communication with patients. It is a fact that almost all CU patients have access to an increasing array of information and communication technologies (ICTs). They regularly use for health information and self-management education (SME).[7]

A timely and challenging objective for clinicians is the use of information technology for patient education while ensuring high-quality care and, most importantly, patient safety. Patients with CU improve their everyday quality of life by receiving complex interventions known as therapeutic patient education (TPE). TPE is a time-intense and expensive process but improves information and abilities for CU patients to deal with skin conditions.[8]

Artificial intelligence (AI) acts as a potentially powerful tool for patient education, especially in recent times.[9] Shortly, AI can provide socially assistive robotics (SAR), an emerging field in human-robot interaction (HRI). SAR aims to help humans to implement and transfer knowledge through electronic social interaction rather than physical interaction. It means that the traditional physical interaction will shift to a new social dimension and medical patient relationship. Arguably, this shift provides new opportunities for innovation and PEM for CU due to its broader, less fixed demarcations. At the same time, it also challenges our HRI approach by integrating a complementary approach, which is inspired by both technology and social interaction aspects, into the treatment of CU.

CONCLUSION

Patients and physicians urge PEM development for CU. Ideally, regardless of the PEM utilized, having access to multiple PEM would greatly benefit patients to choose their preferred method(s). It should be noted that no one technique entirely replaces the traditional face-to-face discussion between provider and patient but can sustain the information knowledge transference. As in many educational processes, multiple PEM techniques and technologies used sequentially or concurrently may offer the best opportunity for comprehension, engagement, and therapy success. Using PEM as a conduit for daily patient question answers instead of supplemental traditional informative material should be implemented. Overall, PEM for CU treatment is a complex topic to conceptualize, but we should support our CU patients in understanding their disease to the best of our abilities.

FURTHER INFORMATION

1. www.uptodate.com/patients
2. https://www.bad.org.uk/for-the-public/patient-information-leaflets/urticaria-and-angioedema
3. https://dermnetnz.org/topics/urticaria-an-overview
4. https://www.allergyuk.org/information-and-advice/conditions-and-symptoms/416-urticaria-hives-and-other-skin-allergy

ONLINE REFERENCES

To access the references of this chapter online, kindly refer to **emedicine360.com** also please follow the instructions mentioned on inside cover.

CHAPTER 20

Urticaria in Elderly

Hassan Mobayed, Nasseer Masoodi, Maryam Al-Nesf

INTRODUCTION

Considerable attention focusing on diseases of the elderly is bestowed; however, the definition of elderly is controversial. World Health Organization defines old age as people above age of 65 years.[1] Sixty-five has been accepted as the age of retirement and eligibility for government welfare benefits in 1935 in the United States of America (USA) as the first social security act, then increased to 67 in 1983.[2] In general, being over 65 years of age is generally acknowledged as being old in many nations. The population healthy aging is defined as extending life expectancy while adding healthy years and is the aim of many governments and societies. However, increased longevity is associated at the same time with experiencing the poor health status of aging presented with a progressive loss of physical, mental, and cognitive integrity. This in turn is resulted in functional impairment and increased susceptibility to morbidity and mortality, which may affect the stability of societies.[3] The observed increases in people living longer result from health care and social improvements; however, aging and age-related disease carry a significant burden accounted for 51.3% of the total diseases.[4]

Older individuals are more susceptible to infections and other noncommunicable diseases, including skin disorders and pruritus, which can be explained by one or combined factors, including immunological, skin, and nervous systems changes.[5-8] The immunological background abnormalities in the elderly are suggested to be related to the impairment of adaptive immune responses[5] due to deficiency in antigen-driven selection processes[7] and exhaustion of immune repertoire.[8] At least five skin and subcutaneous diseases were highlighted and connected to aging.[3] The pruritus and skin disease in the elderly population might be a result of changes in the skin, such as reduction in dermal thickness, mast cells loss in dermal layers, and decreased blood flow from basal and cutaneous compartments; which may allow for the development of new or different phenotypes of known diseases in this senior adult population.[6] Finally, a subclinical neuropathy secondary to degeneration in the elderly with skin itchiness, decreased itch threshold to stimuli, and reduced skin hydration was suggested. Pruritus is estimated to range from 11.5 to 41.3% in the elderly, with a prevalence of current chronic pruritus increased with age from 12.3% (16–30 years) to 20.3% (61–70 years) and can be attributed to many etiologies among which urticaria is not an uncommon diagnosis.[6] Urticaria is studied scarcely in the elderly. The insufficient data in the literature are extended to involve multiple aspects, such as epidemiology, etiopathogenesis, clinical aspects, association with co-morbidities, efficacy and safety profiles of treatments, and management strategies. Moreover, the disease of chronic urticaria (CU) adversely affects the quality of life, such as sleep quality and everyday life habits and activities, and may exacerbate or induce severe disability.[9]

This review is focusing on only limited points pertinent to the elderly that may differ from other populations. The first point of concern is the epidemiology of urticaria in the elderly group of patients. Urticaria is more prevalent at age 20–40 years;[6] however, the prevalence of CU in the elderly was estimated in a study conducted in Brazil, in which 1,598 patients with CU were investigated and showed that 82.5% were adults and 9.4% were from the elderly populations. In the elderly group, chronic spontaneous urticaria (CSU) was nearly equally distributed in both sexes and was characterized by fewer wheals, lower rates of concomitant symptomatic dermographism, lower rates of angioedema, and lower autologous serum skin test (ASST) positivity.[10] Another report suggested that patients aged 40 years and above had a prolonged duration of disease. In the same report, 25% of the patients were in the age group 60–79 years, and 3.4% were ≥80 years.[6]

The prevalence of chronic inducible urticaria (CIndU) among elderly patients received a particular interest in one study. It examined patient with CU, found that 153 (7.7%) were elderly out of the 1,970 studied patients with CU; and 26 elderly patients (17%) were diagnosed with CIndU. Most patients suffered from physical urticarias, and symptomatic dermographism was the most frequent, followed by cold urticaria.[11]

The second point of interest is the diagnostic approach. As in adults, the diagnostic work-up of CSU aims to exclude differential diagnoses and identify triggers of exacerbation or any underlying causes if indicated. As the elderly are prone to a more comorbid and increasing number of prescribed medications than other populations, CSU in the elderly should consider the possibilities of underlying internal pathologies such as infectious, autoimmune, neoplastic diseases, as well as allergic causes.[9] Therefore, physicians should devote special emphasis on these areas by a detailed and systemic anamnesis and focused clinical examination. Furthermore, the laboratory work-up in the elderly should be more focused on excluding any potential underlying medical conditions that may not be considered in other age groups as hematological and organs malignancies and end-organ diseases that may predispose to a picture of CU or pruritus resembling CU.[6,9] In the management approach of elderly patients, physicians should be aware of the differential diagnosis, especially refractory to standard treatment. For example, urticarial vasculitis (UV) is an important differential diagnosis and presents with a painful or burning rash that persists beyond 24 hours and may resolve with residual hyperpigmentation or ecchymosis. Patients with UV may have normal or reduced complements levels (C3, C4) and may occur as a primary disorder or secondary to an underlying autoimmune disorder. Although it is a disease of the middle age group, reports identified elderly cases up to 90 years old with UV.

In some cases, the diagnosis can be confirmed with skin biopsy showing small vessels leukocytoclastic vasculitis, and secondary types due to culprits such as infections and medications should always be considered in the elderly. Additional thoughts of more rare differentials may be worth deliberation, such as lymphoproliferative disease and Schnitzler syndrome that both are known to occur with a mean age group of 50 years and above. Both may manifest with chronic urticarial lesions; however, lesions are sparing the face, difficult to treat with the standard treatment, associated with systemic symptoms such as fever and arthralgia, and high inflammatory markers, and monoclonal paraprotein.[12] The comorbid atopic dermatitis was observed in a single study from Korea to be of a higher prevalence.[13] It may be suggested that the environmental factors and dietary habits may play a role here, and so, medical history and allergen-specific laboratory work-up should be sought.

The final point to focus on the care of urticaria in the elderly population is selecting the treatment options and management plan. Generally, the same guidelines for managing urticaria in adults are applied to the elderly; however, few points should be taken into account in this age group. Polypharmacotherapy, which is very frequent in the elderly due to multiple health conditions, can induce unfavorable side-effects due to pharmacokinetic and pharmacodynamic interactions between different active principles of drugs as well as weaker body to handle medications toxicity due to co-morbidities especially involving the three drug metabolism pathways and organs (liver, gut, and kidneys).[9]

The first-generation antihistamines can induce sedation, impairment of memory, and psychomotor function because they cross the blood-brain barrier. Additionally, these medications have anticholinergic effects, and the known side-effects of such reagents, such as urinary retention, arrhythmias, peripheral vasodilation, and postural hypotension, may be augmented in the elderly age group. Such side-effects should be observed and addressed in the elderly population if this medication was the only option to use for controlling the bothersome refractory urticaria.[14]

Currently, the newer generation nonsedating antihistamines are the best and safest option that can be offered for the elderly to manage the CU; however, the safety profile of the nonsedating antihistamines at higher doses is scarce. Moreover, the efficacy and safety of second-line treatment options have not been assessed in the geriatric population with CU, for which treating CU with corticosteroids and cyclosporine (ciclosporin) in this population must be used with caution and with close monitoring for side effects and toxicity.[9] Additionally, the term nonsedating of the newer generation antihistamines indicates a low tendency to diminish central nervous system (CNS) arousal when taken in therapeutic doses. The newer generations may still have a tendency to cross the brain barrier, still have H_1 receptor occupancy up to 17%, and may produce performance impairment if H_1 receptor occupancy exceeds a certain criterion.[15]

The patients or caregivers should be clearly counseled about these potential side effects. The 2019 American Geriatric Society BEERS criteria recommend avoiding the use of first-generation antihistamines as their clearance is reduced with advanced age, leading to a risk of confusion, dry mouth, constipation, and other anticholinergic effects.[16]

So, newer-generation antihistamines are the preferred option with considering dose adjustment in hepatic or renal dysfunction. Escalation to use the second line or the first generation can be considered with weighing risk-benefits.[12]

In a similar management approach as in adult patients with CU, if high dose nonsedating antihistamine could not control symptoms in the elderly, anti-IgE (omalizumab) should always be considered. An Italian real-life experience evaluated the efficacy and safety of omalizumab in elderly patients with non-sedating H_1-antihistamine–refractory CSU in a real-life setting. The study found that omalizumab is a well-tolerated and effective therapy for elderly patients who failed the usual treatment.[17]

In the end, a good number of limitations in the literature addressing CU in the elderly were observed. These include the nonavailability of the prevalence at different geographical locations and the deficiency of comparison between the different ethnicities. Also, the life expectancy associated with urticaria and other comorbid and the life experience of the different antihistamines and the use of other second-line medications as well as the reported side effects. Longitudinal studies and registries are needed to address this population's characteristics and medical needs. Finally, it seems that the focus of most training and educational programs in the field of allergy is toward the management of pediatrics and adult. At the same time, geriatric specialists follow most geriatric populations with limited referrals to allergy specialty and lack of appropriate training about this special population's health concerns. It may be worth to include geriatric population allergy training in the core curriculum for any allergy/immunology residency and/or fellowship. Vice-versa, training in the geriatric programs should include a specific rotation curriculum in allergy immunology services.

SUMMARY

In summary, CU in the elderly is not an uncommon condition. The care of CU in the elderly requires ruling out multiple differentials, including malignancy and autoimmunity. It may require a multidisciplinary team and the availability of a clinical pharmacist. The treatment should focus on identifying and removing culprits from the patient environment when available and using the least medications with the least side effects and drug interactions to achieve control and reduce polypharmacy. It is always important to consider co-morbidities and recheck drug interactions and toxicity accordingly.

 ONLINE REFERENCES

To access the references of this chapter online, kindly refer to **emedicine360.com** also please follow the instructions mentioned on inside cover.

CHAPTER 21

Urticaria in Pregnancy and Lactation

Emek Kocatürk

INTRODUCTION

Chronic urticaria (CU) is characterized by the appearance of wheals, angioedema, or both for >6 weeks (**Fig. 1**).[1] CU is more common in females than males; chronic spontaneous urticaria (CSU) has a point prevalence in women 1.3% versus 0.8% in men while chronic inducible urticaria shows a female:male ratio of 2:1–3:1.[2,3] It is not only more common in females but also female patients with CU have a higher disease activity, higher rates of angioedema, poorer prognosis, refractoriness to treatment, and longer disease course.[4-8] Despite these, our knowledge on the effect of hormonal conditions on CU is largely lacking and pregnancy constitutes one of these prevalent hormonal conditions. Female CU patients frequently have concerns about the course of urticaria during pregnancy and ask their physicians if they have to quit treatment or if they will require additional medication. A recent multicenter study revealed that CU tends to improve during pregnancy in half of the patients and worsen in one-third of them. Worsening of urticaria was associated with having a mild disease before pregnancy and not being on treatment before pregnancy.[9] These findings stress the importance of proper treatment of CU before and during

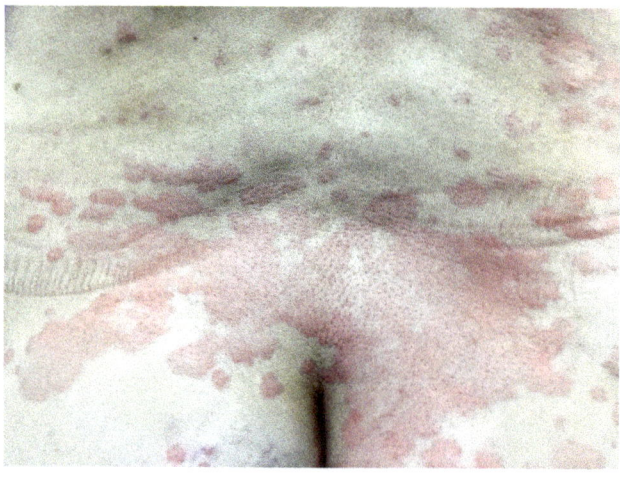

FIG. 1: Chronic urticaria.

pregnancy. Therefore, optimal management of urticaria during pregnancy is vital to ensure the best outcome for the mother and the baby, however, medications' potential risks must be balanced against the effects of untreated disease.

In this chapter, we are going to focus on the treatment of urticaria during pregnancy and lactation.

MANAGEMENT OF URTICARIA DURING PREGNANCY AND LACTATION

Management of CU consists of four major steps: (1) Assessment and monitoring of disease activity; (2) Patient and physician education; (3) Control triggering factors (e.g., physical factors in inducible urticaria, nonsteroidal anti-inflammatory drugs (NSAIDs) in CSU, stress, hot conditions, etc.); (4) Pharmacotherapy.

The key elements of pharmacotherapy are H_1-antihistamines (AHs). The European Academy of Allergology and Clinical Immunology/World Allergy Organization/European Dermatology Forum (EAACI/WAO/EDF) International Urticaria guideline recommends a step-wise approach starting with standard doses of second-generation H_1 AHs, increasing the dose up to four folds in patients who do not respond to standard doses of AHs, adding on omalizumab as the third step and switching to cyclosporine-A in omalizumab nonresponders.[1] In pregnant and lactating patients, the guideline recommends following the same algorithm and emphasizes the lack of knowledge on the safety of urticaria treatment as well as the possible negative effects of increased levels of histamine occurring in urticaria during pregnancy.

Here it would be useful to note that the letter category system of Food and Drug Administration (FDA) on the assignment of pregnancy risk is changing due to the concerns on the application of these letter categories as an oversimplified grading system. A new system is taking place which is called the "Pregnancy and Lactation Labeling Rule" or PLLR.[10] This new system intends to help healthcare providers in evaluating benefit versus risk and in counseling pregnant and nursing patients who need to take medication. This new regulation will eliminate the pregnancy letter categories and will have pregnancy and lactation sections.

H_1-antihistamines

Despite the previously reported associations of both first- and second-generation H_1 AHs with birth defects, detailed analysis of these findings did not provide a meaningful association between AH and major congenital anomalies.[11,12]

Cetirizine and loratadine are the preferred AHs based on their safety data and recommendations in the international urticaria guidelines.[1,13-17] A recent study did not find an association with use of fexofenadine during pregnancy with an increased risk of major birth defects or spontaneous abortion compared with cetirizine use during pregnancy.[18] And use of desloratadine in pregnancy was not associated with a significant increased risk of major birth defects, preterm birth, spontaneous abortion, and small size for gestational age or stillbirth compared with loratadine use in pregnancy.[19]

First-generation H_1 AHs such as chlorpheniramine or diphenhydramine are not recommended as first line agents in the treatment of CU due to their cognitive side effects but might be considered if other options are not working since, they have not been associated with adverse fetal outcomes in prospective cohort trials.[16]

Additionally, the use of H_1 AHs at the first trimester is not associated with increased risk of major malformations or other adverse pregnancy outcomes (spontaneous abortions, prematurity, low-birth weight, and still birth).[20] The pregnancy categories of H_1-AHs are shown in **Table 1**. The safety of higher doses of AHs has not been evaluated in pregnant patients, potential risks and benefits of this treatment should be discussed with the patient before implementing it.

Montelukast

The international guidelines do not recommend the use of leukotriene antagonists for the treatment of CU due to insufficient level of evidence,[1] but if their use is considered during pregnancy, montelukast has been assigned pregnancy category B and no increase in major malformations were reported with the use of montelukast during pregnancy.[21]

Omalizumab

A recombinant immunoglobulin G (IgG1) anti-IgE monoclonal antibody, omalizumab, is the recommended treatment in AH resistant CSU.[1] Animal data (reproduction studies in cynomolgus monkeys) shows no maternal toxicity, impaired male or female fertility, embryotoxicity or teratogenicity, and no adverse effects on fetal or neonatal growth when administered throughout late gestation, delivery and nursing, subcutaneously in doses up to 75 mg/kg (12-fold the maximum clinical dose).[22] Namazy et al. performed a study [the Xolair Pregnancy Registry (EXPECT)] to determine the maternal and neonatal outcomes of female patients with moderate-to-severe asthma treated with conventional drugs and omalizumab (n = 250) during pregnancy and compared with those of a group of asthmatic women treated with conventional drugs but not with omalizumab (n = 1,153). They concluded that they did not detect evidence of an increased risk of major congenital anomalies in the omalizumab-treated group.[23] Since this study includes only asthmatic patients, it is difficult to draw any definitive conclusions for the safety of omalizumab in pregnant females with CU, however, there are 16 case reports on the safe use of omalizumab during pregnancy in CU patients.[24] Considering other options, omalizumab may be a reasonable choice for AH-refractory urticaria during pregnancy. The benefit-risk ratio for treating pregnant women should be reconsidered in every case and it should be kept in mind that since omalizumab has a very long life of elimination half-life (26 days), omalizumab exposure of the neonate would persist for weeks after birth.

Cyclosporine A

Cyclosporine-A is the fourth line treatment in CU treatment guidelines and should be considered in omalizumab nonresponsive patients. It is classified by the FDA as pregnancy risk category "C". The use of calcineurin inhibitors such as cyclosporine during pregnancy does not increase the risk for congenital defects in infants.[25]

A meta-analysis of 15 studies including 410 transplant patients suggested that cyclosporine-A use during pregnancy is not teratogenic but may be associated with low-birth weight in infants (<2,500 g) and premature delivery.[26] Cyclosporine A is generally not recommended in pregnancy since its side-effects such as hypertension and nephrotoxicity can potentiate gestational complications such as pre-eclampsia. It should only be considered after other modalities have failed.[27]

Systemic Steroids

The guidelines recommend the use of systemic steroids only during exacerbations of CU for short periods. In general, steroids are not considered to be teratogenic, but fetal exposure to systemic steroids (median 20 mg/day) during intrauterine development has been linked to growth retardation.[28] A meta-analysis showed an increased risk of approximately three-folds for oral clefts.[29] However, a case–control study from United States National Birth Defects Prevention showed no increased risk for oral clefts with first trimester systemic steroid use.[30] Systemic corticosteroid use in pregnancy may lead to maternal adverse effects such as hypertension, preeclampsia, and gestational diabetes and these can negatively affect fetal outcomes (i.e., intrauterine growth restriction, intrauterine fetal demise, and macrosomia). Therefore, systemic steroids should be avoided in pregnancy if possible, if used, must be prescribed at the lowest effective dose of ≤20 mg/day of prednisone for severe, recalcitrant cases for a limited period of time.[31,32] Short courses of 1–5 days during exacerbations (minimum effective dose and shortest duration) are unlikely to cause pregnancy complications. Prednisone and methylprednisolone are the steroids of choice (FDA category B); since due to their short half-life they are effectively metabolized by 11-β-hydroxy-steroid which is present in the placenta and fetal exposure is approximately 10% of the maternal plasma level.[33-35]

TREATMENT DURING LACTATION

Antihistamines

Second-generation AHs are safe to use during lactation since the transfer rate to breast milk is minimal.[36] Loratadine, cetirizine, and fexofenadine are the best studied AHs.[37,38] First-generation AHs might lead to infant irritability and drowsiness,[39] therefore, second-generation AHs should be preferred. Higher doses of loratadine and terfenadine showed very minimal transmission to the milk.[34,40] Hence, the transfer rate to breast-milk is minimal, in refractory cases of CU who are nursing their babies, higher doses of second-generation AHs can be safely used.[34]

Systemic Steroids

The American Academy of Pediatrics consider systemic steroids safe to use during lactation and recommend prednisone or prednisolone over other options.[41] But infant exposure should be limited to the lowest effective dose for the shortest duration. Studies have shown low amounts of prednisolone can be transferred to breast milk; which represents <10% of the infant's endogenous cortisol level.[42] It is recommended to wait to breastfeed 4 hours after maternal ingestion to avoid peak plasma levels occurring 1 hour after ingestion.[43]

Montelukast

Montelukast levels in breast milk are very low and it is approved for use in children as young as 6 months of age. Therefore, amounts ingested by infants during breastfeeding are not expected to cause any adverse effects.[44] A task force of respiratory experts from Australia, New Zealand, and Europe found that these drugs are probably safe during breastfeeding.[45]

Omalizumab

Since omalizumab is a large protein molecule, with a molecular weight of 145,058 Da, it is likely that omalizumab levels in milk are very low. It is supposed to be partially destroyed in the gastrointestinal tract of the infant and systemic absorption by the infant is probably minimal.[46] The EXPECT pregnancy registry has followed pregnant and nursing females for several years and 154 infants were breastfed while their mothers were on omalizumab treatment. No difference in serious adverse events were seen among the infants who received or did not receive omalizumab. Infections occurred at a similar rate in all groups.[23] In a recent case report, a pregnant CU patient was treated with omalizumab and continued to receive it while nursing the infant. The authors reported that approximately 1/10,000 to 1/1,000 of omalizumab in maternal serum is transferred into human breast milk.[47]

Cyclosporine A

Cyclosporine A treated mother's breastfed infant would usually receive often <1% of the mother's weight-adjusted dosage. No adverse effects on infant's growth, development or kidney function have been reported. Breastfed infants should be monitored if cyclosporine-A is used during lactation, including measurement of serum cyclosporine levels to rule out toxicity.[48]

See **Table 1** for pregnancy and lactation considerations for medications used for the treatment of CU.

TABLE 1: Pregnancy and lactation considerations for medications used for the treatment of chronic urticaria.

Medication	Pregnancy considerations	Lactation considerations
Cetirizine	PLLR is available (https://pdf.hres.ca/dpd_pm/00035506.PDF)	Excretion in breast-milk is considered low
Loratadine	PLLR is available (https://omr.bayer.ca/omr/online/claritin-pm-en.pdf)	Excretion in breast-milk is considered low
Chlorpheniramine	PLLR is available (https://www.accessdata.fda.gov/drugsatfda_docs/nda/2015/206323Orig1s000Lbl.pdf)	Excretion in breast-milk is not known
Hydroxyzine	PLLR is available. In product monograph contraindicated in early (first trimester) pregnancy (http://eci2012.net/wp-content/uploads/2015/03/Atarax-En-Monograph-100902.04-Jan-2015.pdf)	Excretion in breast-milk is not known. May cause drowsiness in newborn
Diphenhydramine	Pregnancy category B	Excretion in breast-milk is considered low. May cause drowsiness in newborn

Continued

Continued

Medication	Pregnancy considerations	Lactation considerations
Montelukast	Pregnancy category B	Excretion in breast-milk is considered low
Omalizumab	PLLR is available (https://www.novartis.ca/sites/www.novartis.ca/files/xolair_scrip_e.pdf)	Excretion in breast-milk is considered very low
Systemic corticosteroids	Pregnancy category B (for prednisolone and methylprednisolone)	Excretion in breast-milk is considered very low
Cyclosporine	Pregnancy category C	Excretion in breast-milk is considered low. Detectable in infant's blood

(PLLR: pregnancy and lactation labeling rule)

CONCLUSION

Pregnant CU patients should be informed about the course of the disease that there may be exacerbations and no-treatment could end-up with emergency referrals and worsening of the disease during pregnancy. Even though, the ideal situation during pregnancy and lactation is "no pharmacologic therapy", especially during the first trimester, it is almost impossible for a CU patient to have no disease activity during pregnancy. Therefore, the aim of treatment of CU during pregnancy is to have zero or minimal disease activity with the least possible treatment. The potential side effects of any drug must be balanced against the risks to the mother or the infant against inadequately treated disease.

USEFUL LINKS

And besides the FDA categories we can also check if there is pregnancy registry studies for the relevant drug (https://www.fda.gov/science-research/womens-health-research/list-pregnancy-exposure-registries).
For lactation database visit the Drugs and Lactation Database (LactMed) [Internet]. https://www.ncbi.nlm.nih.gov/books/NBK501922/

 ONLINE REFERENCES

To access the references of this chapter online, kindly refer to **emedicine360.com** also please follow the instructions mentioned on inside cover.

CHAPTER 22

Urticaria in Kidney Disease, Liver Disease, and Cardiac Disease

Carla Ritchie

INTRODUCTION

This chapter describes the characteristics of chronic spontaneous urticaria (CSU) in different special situations such as urticaria in kidney, liver, and cardiac disease.

URTICARIA IN KIDNEY DISEASE

Pruritus is the most common cutaneous complaint in patients with chronic renal failure. Although uremic pruritus etiology is not known, several hypothesis have been proposed: Mastocites and histamine, parathormone, ions (Ca, P, and Mg), xerosis, hypervitaminosis A, neuropathy, membranes biocompatibility and dialysis efficacy, and psychosomatic. Chronic urticaria (CU) is not one of the most common diseases in patients with chronic kidney failure.[1]

However, CU was significantly associated with chronic renal failure, in a study conducted to evaluate the association of CU and metabolic syndrome (MS).[2]

Treatment of Chronic Urticaria in Kidney Disease

Second-generation antihistamines are the drugs of choice as the first line in the treatment of CU due to their safety and efficacy profile.[3] The absorption, distribution, metabolism, and elimination processes of these antihistamines were evaluated in different populations such as healthy subjects, in the elderly, and also in patients with kidney or liver diseases.[4]

Knowledge of the pharmacokinetics of antihistamines is the key to their correct use in special populations such as patients with kidney disease, especially with regard to drug interactions. Drugs that are poorly metabolized have a lower risk of drug interactions when administered with other drugs.[5]

Second-generation Antihistamines

- *Bilastine*: In the case of bilastine, studies have been carried out to evaluate the effect of renal insufficiency in terms of pharmacokinetics. In patients with renal failure, an increase in the plasma concentration of the drug is observed that is not related to changes in the safety margin of the drug.[6]

  Since bilastine is a substrate for P-glycoprotein (P-gp), the concomitant administration of drugs or foods capable of inhibiting P-gp should be avoided in patients with moderate or severe disease.[6]

- *Desloratadine*: Caution suggested in severe renal impairment (RI)[4]
- *Ebastine*: It is not necessary to change the dose in patients with RI[7]
- *Fexofenadine*: No dose adjustment necessary[4]
- *Cetirizine*: There are no clinical data to document the efficacy/safety relationship in patients with renal insufficiency. As cetirizine is mainly eliminated via the kidneys in cases where that an alternative treatment cannot be used, the intervals of dosage according to renal function. The elimination half-life of cetirizine was evaluated in a study involving 30 healthy subjects of different ages and 15 patients with renal failure with different stages of severity. An increase in the elimination half-life of cetirizine and a reduction in renal clearance were observed.[7,8] In turn, in another study, multiple doses of cetirizine were administered in patients on hemodialysis and it was concluded that a dose of 5 mg three times a week was an adequate and safe dose for these types of patients.[9]
- *Levocetirizine*: The technical file recommends adjusting the dosage intervals in the case of RI. Contraindicated in severe RI[4]
- *Rupatadine*: No studies are available on rupatadine in patients with RI. At present its use is not recommended in this type of patients[4]

URTICARIA IN LIVER DISEASE

In a recent review by Kocatürk et al.[10] they conducted a literature search on the relationship between urticaria and liver.

The data found were few. We describe a case report of a 25-year-old young man with a history of cholinergic urticaria who presented signs of cellular liver injury in the cholinergic urticarial crises.[11]

Other case reports of patients with yellow urticaria are also mentioned, in patients with different liver diseases and high levels of bilirubin. This particularity could be related to the increase in vascular permeability in urticaria, which would generate the exudation of bilirubin into urticarial hives.[12]

Treatment of Chronic Urticaria in Liver Disease

There are few reports that associate the use of antihistamines and hepatotoxicity. Rare cases of acute liver injury have been reported, which are generally mild and self-limiting conditions.[13]

In recent years, isolated cases of hepatotoxicity have been described with the use of different second-generation antihistamines, such as mizolastine,[14] terfenadine,[15] and ebastine[16] or even more serious reactions, such as subfulminant liver failure with loratadine[17] or severe and recurrent hepatitis with use of cetirizine.[18,19] The triggering mechanism for this reaction by the different antihistamines is unknown.

URTICARIA AND CARDIAC DISEASE

Same studies have found that hypertension is associated with an extended and severity duration of CU.

In a prospective study of 228 patients with moderate-to-severe CU, a correlation was observed between the presence of systemic hypertension and more persistent symptoms. Among hypertensive patients, resolution was seen in 19 and 26% at

2 and 5 years, respectively, compared with 37 and 46% in patients with normal pressure. The duration of urticaria would not be related to the different types of antihypertensive drugs.[20] In one cohort, it was described that patients with urticaria had a 1.37 times greater risk of developing hypertension than controls. And that this risk would probably be related to alterations in the coagulation and fibrinolysis cascades. In the same way preliminary evidence from the limited data currently available.[21]

In the same sense, data from recent studies seem to support the relationship between CSU and MS. The presence of MS would be related to a different endotype of urticaria, in the nonautoreactive forms. In turn, it would behave as an independent risk factor for more severe forms with less response to treatment. One of the theories that explain it is the presence of a constant inflammatory state in the MS.

Metabolic syndrome and CSU will share some pathophysiological mechanisms such as proinflammatory status, increased oxidative stress, activation in the coagulation cascade, and alterations in the adipokine profile.[22]

Metabolic syndrome and its components increase the risk of ischemic heart disease, myocardial infarction and stroke, leading to reduced life quality and expectancy.[23]

Treatment of Chronic Urticaria and Cardiac Disease

As mentioned previously in this chapter, the drugs of first choice for the treatment of CU are second-generation antihistamines. Many patients do not respond to the usual doses and, following the recommendations of the Global Allergy and Asthma European Network (GALEN) guidelines,[3] they should even quadruple their dose. It is important to evaluate the safety when the doses are used in a way greater than the licensed doses, being a key aspect in the study of the safety are possible cardiotoxic effects.

A recent review on cardiotoxicity and second-generation antihistamines used in unlicensed doses has concluded that these drugs have an excellent safety profile, with no evidence of cardiotoxicity. They studied in detail bilastine, cetirizine, levocetirizine, ebastine, fexofenadine, loratadine, desloratadine, mizolastine, and rupatadine.

These conclusions nonetheless emphasize that whenever doctors who indicate these drugs, especially in unusual doses, previously evaluate certain risk factors such as the presence of long QT syndrome, advanced age, cardiovascular disorders, hypokalemia, and hypomagnesemia, or the use of drugs that have direct QT-prolonging effects or inhibit the metabolism of antihistamines.[24]

 ONLINE REFERENCES

To access the references of this chapter online, kindly refer to **emedicine360.com** also please follow the instructions mentioned on inside cover.

Index

Page numbers followed by *b* refer to box, *f* refer to figure, *fc* refer to flowchart, and *t* refer to table.

A

Absorption 66
Acrivastine 66
Activity impairment score 73
Acute allergic urticaria 11
Acute febrile neutrophilic dermatosis 50
Acute nonallergic urticaria 9
Acute spontaneous urticaria 69
Acute urticaria 3, 9, 5*f*, 10*b*, 12, 48, 50, 88, 89, 105
   differential diagnosis of 50
Adalimumab 80
Adrenaline 12, 53
Aggravating chronic spontaneous urticaria 15
Allergic diseases 38, 41
Allergy 38
Alpha-galactosidase anaphylaxis 11
Aluminum 67
Anaphylaxis 38, 50
Ancylostoma 7
Anemia, pernicious 39, 40
Angioedema 9, 13, 16, 31, 33-34, 44, 44*f*, 47, 50, 52, 53, 55, 62
   acquired 34
   activity score 58, 62, 63, 91
   control test 62, 64, 91
   cyclic episodes of 52
   differential diagnosis of 52
   episodic 52
   etiologies of 34*f*
   hereditary 34, 36, 53
   mast cell mediated 53
   quality of life questionnaire 62
   recurrent 53*b*, 62
   vibratory 27
Angiotensin-converting enzyme 34
   inhibitor 35, 53, 55
      pathogenesis of 97

Anisakis simplex 7, 10, 16, 40
   anaphylaxis 11
Antacids 67
Antialpha adrenergic effects 65
Antibody
   antineutrophil cytoplasmic 51
   antinuclear 15, 39, 51
   monoclonal 98
Anticholinergic effects 65
Anticoagulants 80, 82
Antihistamines 33, 53, 65-67, 91, 108, 117
   classification of 65, 66
   nonsedating 67, 69
Anti-immunoglobulin E 79, 85
Antiserotoninergic effects 65
Anti-thyroidperoxidase 98
Anti-tumor necrosis factor 77
   alpha 80, 99
Anxiety 16, 57
Aquagenic urticaria 2, 24, 26, 30
Asthma 8, 38
Atopic diseases 9
Atopy 8
Autoallergic reaction 5
Autoantibodies 14, 96
Autoimmune
   diseases 8, 38
   hypothyroidism 54
   progesterone dermatitis 52
   thyroid disease 17, 38
Autoimmunity 14, 15, 38, 39
Autoinflammatory diseases 51
Autologous blood injection 80, 82
Autologous plasma skin test 58
Autologous serum skin test 2, 15, 18, 39, 58, 97, 111
Autosomal dominant disorder 53
Axon reflex 3
Azathioprine 80, 83
Azelastine 67, 68

B

Bacteria 7
Basopenia 14
Basophil 14
   activation test 2, 15, 18
   histamine release assay 2, 15, 39
Benralizumab 98
Bepotastine 67
Bilastine 66-68, 85, 120
Blastocystis hominis 7, 40
Blood 96
   biochemistry 51
   test 58
   vessels 96
Body temperature 107
Bradykinin-mediated angioedema 35, 53
   treatments for 37
Brain 66
Breastfeeding 108
Breath, shortness of 9
British Association of Dermatologists 104
Bronchodilators 33
Bruton's tyrosine kinase 100
   inhibitor 23, 100
Bullous pemphigoid 18, 38, 52
Burning 56

C

Cardiac disease 120-122
Cardiovascular disease 41
Celiac disease 39, 40
Cellulitis 18, 53
Central nervous system 66, 112
Cetirizine 66-68, 115, 118, 121
Cheilitis, granulomatous 53
Chemokines 3
Children's dermatology life quality index 91
Chlamydia pneumonia 40, 46
Chloroquine 80, 82
Chlorpheniramine 118
   maleate 66
Cholinergic urticaria 2, 13, 24, 25, 28, 28f, 90, 100
Chronic idiopathic urticaria 38, 72
Chronic inducible urticaria 1, 2, 7, 13, 24, 27, 49, 58, 61, 75, 85, 87-89, 111
Chronic spontaneous urticaria 1, 2, 8, 13, 14-19, 19b, 23, 31, 34, 45, 48, 56, 60, 70, 72, 74, 85, 88, 88f, 89, 98, 99, 101, 103, 108, 111, 114, 120
   autoimmune etiology of 38
   cellular components of 14
   clinical trials 73
   differential diagnosis of 18b
Chronic urticaria 1, 3, 5f, 13, 17, 48, 55, 61, 70, 74, 79, 80, 80t, 84, 88, 98, 101, 103, 105, 106, 111, 114, 114f, 118t, 120
   classification of 2t
   differential diagnosis of 50
   pathogenesis of 101f
   quality life questionnaire 60, 62, 73
   subtypes 2
   treatment of 79, 84fc, 101, 120-122
Cimetidine 80, 81
Clemastine 84
Cold 107
   provocation test 90f
   urticaria 2, 24, 25, 28f, 29, 89, 90f
Complete blood count 51, 58
Connective tissue disease 51
Contact urticaria 2, 27, 31
Coronavirus disease-2019 10, 44
   pandemic 40
Corticosteroids 80, 83
   systemic 119
COVID-19 10, 44
   infection 40, 46
      cutaneous manifestations of 46
   outbreak 46
   pandemic 40
   vaccinations 45
Coxsackie A9 virus 10, 45
C-reactive protein 15, 51, 58
Cryopyrin-associated periodic syndromes 51
Cyclosporine 21, 92, 119
   A 70, 116, 118
   response 8
Cytokines 3
Cytomegalovirus 10, 45, 58

D

Dapsone 21, 80
Darier's sign 52f
D-chlorpheniramine 67
Delayed pressure urticaria 2, 13, 24, 25, 29
Dental infections 7
Deoxyribonucleic acid 81
   double stranded 15, 97
Depression 16
Dermatitis
   allergic contact 54
   atopic 17, 70
   urticarial 52

Dermatology life quality index 32, 73
Dermatomyositis 54
Dermatosis, progesterone-induced 18
Dermographic urticaria 27
Dermographism, symptomatic 24, 27, 28f, 89, 90f
Desloratadine 66, 68, 121
Diabetes mellitus 39
   insulin-dependent 38, 40
Diarrhea 9, 11
Diphenhydramine 66, 67, 118
Dizziness 9
Doxepin 66, 80, 81
Drugs 10, 16, 106
Dupilumab 23, 80, 99
Dyspnea 9, 11

E

Ebastine 66-68, 121
Ecchymosis 56
Edema 56
Enzyme-linked immunosorbent assay 15
Eosinopenia 14
Eosinophilia 52
Eosinophilic cellulitis 54
Eosinophils 14, 98
Epinastine 67
Epinephrine 12, 53
   intramuscular 33
Epstein–Barr virus 10, 46, 58
Erysipelas 18, 53
Erythema 56
   annulare centrifugum 52
   marginatum 36
   multiforme 18, 50
Erythrocyte sedimentation rate 27, 51
Erythromycin 67
Etanercept 80
European Academy of Allergology and Clinical Immunology 1, 20, 44, 60, 72, 91, 115
European Dermatology Forum 1, 20, 44, 60, 72, 115
Exercise 107

F

Fever 52
Fexofenadine 66-68, 85, 121
Figurate erythemas 18
First generation antihistamines 65, 66, 69
   classification of 66t

Fluids, intravenous 33
Folic acid antagonist 81
Food
   allergies 106
   anaphylaxis, exercise-induced 11
Fragment crystallizable epsilon receptor 1 95, 101

G

Gammapathy, monoclonal 34
Gastroenterology 56
Gastroesophageal reflux disease, prevalence of 17
Gastrointestinal disorders 38
Gleich syndrome 52
Global Allergy and Asthma European Network 1, 20, 44, 60, 72, 122
Glomerular filtration rate 68
Glucocorticoids 53
Glycoprotein 68
G-protein coupled receptors 65
Graft versus host disease 70
Granulocyte-macrophage colony-stimulating factor 95
Graves' disease 39, 40

H

H_1-antihistamine
   less-sedating 67
   pharmacokinetics of 66
   sedating 67
   selection of 69
Hansen disease 18
Hashimoto's thyroiditis 39
Headache 9
Heat urticaria 2, 24, 26, 30
Helicobacter pylori 7, 16, 27, 40, 44, 46, 58
   infection 46
Henoch–Schönlein purpura 17, 39
Heparin sodium 80
Hepatitis 51
   A 7, 10
      viruses 45
   acute 58
   B 7, 40
      infection 17, 45
      virus 10, 17, 45
   C 7, 40
      infection 17, 45
      virus 17, 45
Herpes simplex virus 7, 10

Histamine 3, 65, 120
Human basophils 45
Human herpesvirus 46
Human immunodeficiency virus 7, 51
Human leukocyte antigen 39
Human-robot interaction 108
Hydroxychloroquine 80, 82
Hydroxyzine 66, 67, 84, 118
Hyperpigmentation, postinflammatory 51
Hypersensitivity 4
Hypertension 85
Hypervitaminosis A 120
Hypocomplementemic urticarial vasculitis syndrome 51
Hypotension, arterial 11

I

Ice cube test 90f
Idiopathic nonmast cell angioedema 37
Immunoglobulin E 14, 16, 23, 38, 50, 58, 95
   autoantibodies 8
   mediated urticaria 4
Immunoglobulin G 8
   autoantibodies 8
   mediated urticaria 5
Immunoglobulin
   intravenous 21, 80, 82
   subcutaneous 80
Inducible urticaria 8, 105, 115
   features of 24t
   treatment of 31
Infections 9, 10, 15, 38, 106
   chronic viral 17, 40
Inflammatory bowel disease 17, 39
Infliximab 80
Insect
   bites 50
   stings 106
Interferon 21
   gamma 70
Interleukin 15, 23, 70, 101
Itching 56

J

Janus kinase inhibitor 80

K

Kallikrein–Kinin pathways 36
Kawasaki disease 17, 39
Ketoconazole 67

Ketotifen 67
Kidney 120
   disease 120
   impairment 68

L

Lactation 114, 115, 118t
Leukocytes 96
Leukotrienes 3, 4
   receptor antagonists 21
   synthesis 4
Levocetirizine 66-68, 121
Ligelizumab 23, 99
Lips, angioedema of 10f
Livedo reticularis 56
Liver 120
   disease 120, 121
   impairment 68
Long QT-syndrome 85
Loratadine 67, 68, 118
Low-grade systemic inflammatory disease 39
Lymphocytes 14

M

Maculopapular cutaneous mastocytosis 52, 52f
Magnesium 67
Malaise 11
Malassezia globosa 7
Mast cell 6, 14, 34, 38, 95
   activation mechanisms 4
   angioedema 33
   cutaneous 14
   degranulation 95
   diseases 99
   driven disease 3
   independent urticaria 97
   receptors 4f
   stimulating factors of 95f
Mepolizumab 80, 98
Mequitazine 67
Metabolic syndrome 38, 41, 120
Methotrexate 21, 80, 81
Mizolastine 66, 68
Monoamine oxidase inhibitors 66
Montelukast 21, 80, 116, 117, 119
   inhibits 79
Mood disorders 57
Mycobacterium leprae 46
Mycophenolate mofetil 80, 81
Mycoplasma pneumonia 7, 10, 40, 45, 46

N

Nausea 9
Nephrotic syndrome 70
Nerves 96
Neuropathy 120
Nonphysical chronic inducible urticaria 90
Nonphysical urticarias 24
Nonsteroidal anti-inflammatory drugs 5, 8, 10, 16, 41, 50, 56, 115
    reactions 8
Normocomplementemic urticarial vasculitis 51

O

Occupational contact urticaria 57
Olopatadine 67
Omalizumab 7, 20, 72, 74-78, 85, 92, 116, 118, 119
    response 8
    treatment 87
Oral corticosteroids 22, 84
Oral steroids 108

P

Pain, abdominal 9, 11, 50
Palmoplantar pruritus 11
Parainfluenza viruses 45
Parasites 7
Parathormone 120
Parvovirus B19 10
Patient education materials 103, 104
    assessment tool 104
    function 104
    models 104
Pemphigoid gestationis 52
Pharmacotherapy 115
Phototherapy 21
Physical chronic inducible urticaria 89
Plasma protein binding 67
Plasmapheresis 21, 80, 82
Plasmodium falciparum 10
Polymorphic light eruption 50
Postlesion hyperpigmentation 56
Prednisolone 12
Pregnancy 108, 114, 115, 118*t*
    and lactation labeling rule 119
Pressure 107
Promethazine 66
Prostaglandin 3, 14
Pruritus 56, 120
Pseudoallergen-free diet 80, 81
Psoriasis 39, 40, 70
Psychiatric
    diseases 42
    disorders 38

R

Randomized controlled trials 20, 73, 81, 91
Ranitidine 80, 81
Rapid eye movement 66
    sleep 66
Raynaud phenomena 56
Reflex erythema 49
Refractory chronic spontaneous urticarial, treatment of 22
Refractory uveitis 70
Renal toxicity 85
Reslizumab 98
Rheumatoid
    arthritis 38-40, 70
    factor 51
Rhinitis, allergic 17, 69
Rhinovirus 7
Rifampin 67
Rituximab 99
Rotavirus 7
Rupatadine 66, 67, 121
Ruxolitinib 80

S

Schistosoma mansoni 7, 40
Schnitzler syndrome 51
Sclerosis
    amyotrophic lateral 70
    multiple 38
Second generation antihistamines 15, 66, 79, 84, 120
    advantages of 68
    classification of 66*t*
    use of 68*t*
Secukinumab 99
Serum creatinine 51
Shock, anaphylactic 11
Sinusitis, recurrent 47
Sjögren's syndrome 39, 54
Skeeters syndrome 57
Skin
    biopsy 107
    patch test 58
Solar urticaria 2, 24, 29, 30
Somatoform disorders 16
Spleen tyrosin kinase 100
Staphylococcus aureus 45
Steroids, systemic 117
Streptococcal infection 45
Stress, emotional 16, 38, 42

Strongyloides 7
   stercoralis 10
Sulfasalazine 21, 80, 81
Sunlight 107
Sweating 11, 107
Sweet's syndrome 50
Systemic lupus erythematosus 18, 39

T

Tachycardia 65
Tacrolimus 80
Terfenadine 67
T-helper cells 14
Therapeutic patient education 22, 108
Thymic stromal lymphopoietin 100
Thyroglobulin 15
Thyroid function test 58
Thyroperoxidase 5, 15
Tissue factor 15
Tolypocladium inflatum 70
Tonsillitis 47
Topical spleen tyrosine kinase inhibitor 100
Toxic erythema 18
Tranexamic acid 80, 82
Trauma 57
Tumor necrosis factor 80, 95
   alpha 3, 23, 70, 101

U

Ultraviolet light 80, 81
Upper respiratory tract infections 9
Urinary retention 65
Urinary tract infections 7
Urticaria 1, 3, 4, 10, 13, 16, 38-42, 44, 44*f*, 46-48, 55, 58*fc*, 69, 88, 94, 104, 105*f*, 108, 110, 114, 120, 121
   activity score 18, 60, 73, 86, 91
   causes of 105
   classification 1
   control test 32, 58, 60, 61, 74, 91
   diagnosis of 18, 98
   diagnostic approach of 55, 56
   factitia 27
   management of 115
   mechanism of 96
   pathogenesis of 4*f*, 14, 94, 94*fc*
   treatment of 98
   types of 97, 105
Urticarial vasculitis 18, 51, 111
   lesions of 52*f*
Uterine cramps 50

V

Vasculitis, experimental 38
Vibratory urticaria 2, 24, 32
Viral exanthem 50
Viral infection 46, 51
Vitiligo 17, 39, 40
Vomiting 11, 50

W

Weight gain 52
Wells syndrome 54
Western blot 15
Work impairment score 73
World Allergy Organization 1, 20, 44, 60, 72, 115

X

Xerosis 120

Y

Yersinia enterocolitica 40

EU GSPR Authorised Reprsentative
Logos Europe, 9 rue Nicolas Poussin
1700, La Rochelle, France
Phone: +33 (0) 6 67 93 73 78
E-mail: contact@logoseurope.eu

www.ingramcontent.com/pod-product-compliance
Ingram Content Group UK Ltd.
Pitfield, Milton Keynes, MK11 3LW, UK
UKHW050703160426
5217IPUK00041B/1296